SURVIVE!

SURVIVE!

An Emergency Preparedness and Survival Guide

I. M. Reddy

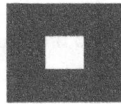

Blue Peter Enterprises, LLC
Dayton, Ohio

Survival Series

Published by
Blue Peter Enterprises, LLC
Dayton, Ohio

Library of Congress Catalog Number 2012932894

ISBN 978-0-9851481-0-2

Disclaimer

The information in this book is intended for general information purposes only; it is not intended to replace advice and expertise from trained professionals. Neither the author nor the publisher is engaged in rendering legal, accounting, tax, medical, or other professional services. The author and the publisher do not warrant the accuracy, completeness, safety, efficacy, or usefulness of the information, text, graphics, or other items in this book. Neither the author nor the publisher advocates the use of any particular drug, chemical, equipment, or procedure mentioned in this book. Neither the author nor the publisher is responsible for any loss, injury, or damage caused as a result of the use, proper or improper, of the information in this book, or for any prosecution or proceeding brought against any person or body that may result from using the information in this book. The reader is solely responsible for the use of the information contained in this book and the results obtained from such use.

Neither the author nor the publisher is responsible for the content available on any Internet web site, including, without limitation, outdated, inaccurate, or incomplete information, and access to any site is at the user's own risk.

Nothing in this book should be construed or interpreted to infringe on the rights of others or to violate criminal statutes. The reader is solely responsible for obeying laws and respecting other people's rights and property.

To Shelby

Failure to prepare is preparing to fail.

~ Benjamin Franklin

This book is about self-reliance. It's about learning to take care of yourself and your loved ones with minimal help from authorities. Unlike some other publications about survival, it's not about feeding your fear; it's about giving you peace of mind. To become a "prepper" or a survivalist, it's not necessary to slip into a siege mentality. In fact, it's important not to. Worry makes your life miserable. Preparedness makes you confident.

The kinds of calamities that can affect our lives are wide-ranging: heat waves, droughts, dust storms, mudslides, rockslides, sinkholes, volcanoes, blizzards, avalanches, floods, earthquakes, tsunamis, hurricanes, tornadoes, epidemics, famine, brownouts, blackouts, explosions, fires, chemical spills, nuclear meltdowns, hijackings, workplace violence, civil unrest, terrorist attacks, financial collapse, infrastructure breakdowns...and more. Disasters may be natural, man-made, or some combination of the two. They may be accidental or deliberate.

Even though you may not be near one of these events when it happens, it can still have a dramatic effect on you.

▶ A 9.2 magnitude earthquake in Alaska in 1964 was felt around the world. It sank several fishing boats in Louisiana, and tsunamis triggered by the quake caused damage in Hawaii and Japan. Aftershocks were felt for 18 months.

▶ The failure to trim trees around power lines in Ohio caused the Northeast Blackout of 2003, a widespread power outage that affected 55 million people in eight U.S. states and Ontario, Canada. Homes and businesses were without power for two days.

▶ In late August, 2008, Hurricane Ike started as a tropical disturbance near Africa. It worked its way across the Atlantic Ocean, and on September 13th, struck the Gulf Coast of the United States. On September 14th, the remnants of the storm created high winds that caused widespread damage and power outages that lasted for 12 days in some areas of the Midwest.

Preface

What's going to happen next? No one can say what, or when, or where. But the earth is a volatile, living planet. The earth's continental plates are moving, as they always have, and those movements cause earthquakes and tsunamis. The earth has experienced natural phenomena such as volcanoes, hurricanes, and tornadoes for thousands of years, and in all likelihood these geological and meteorological events are going to continue. And we certainly don't have any immunity against hostilities from our fellow man. Humans have been waging war against each other for thousands of years. People fight over land and natural resources such as oil, water, lumber, and food. They fight over religion. They fight over power. Our planet is projected to have 9 billion people by the year 2050. Think we're going to stop killing each other? It's probably a safe bet that we won't. When conflicts are so big that they're called "world wars" and when they happen so often that they have to be numbered, it's obvious that humans have some serious issues with one another.

Between changing weather patterns, the strain of rising population on our infrastructure and resources, and the increasingly unstable political situations in the world, the likelihood that you will be the victim of some disaster, whether natural or man-made, is increasing. But the point is not to be afraid; the point is to prepare. We can do little to prevent big disasters, so it serves no purpose to worry about them. But we can control how we react to them.

You may think that in case of a major disaster, the "authorities" are going to handle the situation and "they" will take care of you. Here are some examples of how well your elected officials and their appointees, people paid with your tax dollars, have performed:

▶ During the 1979 meltdown at the Three Mile Island nuclear facility, government officials and the utility company released false and contradictory statements about the release of radiation into the atmosphere.

▶ The Chicago Heat Wave of 1995 killed more than 700 people over a five-day period, yet city officials didn't issue a heat emergency warning until the last day. The city's cooling centers were underutilized, and medical facilities were overwhelmed. So many people died in such a short period of time that the coroner had to use refrigerated trucks to store the bodies, yet some officials denied a problem existed.

▶ Hurricane Katrina blew through New Orleans in 2005, leaving over 1,800 people confirmed dead and more than 700 missing. The Army Corps of Engineers was widely criticized for the poor design of the levees that resulted in the deaths of so many people, and other federal, state, and local agencies were widely criticized for their gross mismanagement of rescue and recovery in the aftermath.

Corporations perform no better. After the Deepwater Horizon oil rig explosion, it was discovered that BP's emergency response manual listed a Professor Peter Lutz as a national wildlife expert, someone to be consulted in case of an oil spill. Unfortunately, Professor Lutz had been dead for four years. What good is an emergency response plan if no one keeps it up to date?

History shows us that no matter the kind of disaster, no matter the decade, the authorities, public or private, can't always be counted on for help. How is it that we can put a man on the moon with a slide rule, but we can't figure out how to save people when we have sufficient warning of an impending disaster? This may happen for several reasons.

One is that the knowledge gained from past experience is known by only a few individuals within the organization. "Tribal knowledge" is lost when people leave the organization. Sometimes organizations purposely don't record events in order to reduce the risk that their incompetence, errors in judgment, or other mistakes might be revealed outside of the organization, with political, legal, or financial ramifications.

Another reason is disagreement between government agencies and levels of government about who is responsible. Six months after Hurricane Ike roared through Texas in 2008, over 300 businesses still had not been paid for their emergency response services, some of them for basic items such as portable showers and toilets. State officials expected the federal government to pay the vendors directly, while federal officials expected the state to pay the vendors and then seek reimbursement from the federal government. The end result is that these vendors may be reluctant to provide services in the future until they have assurances they'll be paid in a timely manner. So instead of past experience making emergency response better the next time around, it may be worse. (If you're there when the next disaster hits Texas, good luck finding a toilet!)

Another reason is that in the face of a widespread catastrophe, officials and volunteers may simply become overwhelmed. Look at the triple disasters that struck Japan in 2011: an earthquake triggered a tsunami that in turn led to a nuclear meltdown. First responders can react to only so many crises before they simply run out of personnel, equipment, and supplies.

Do authorities ever successfully handle a crisis? Of course they do. But you never know beforehand whether a catastrophe will be handled well or poorly. That's why you need to prepare to take care of yourself.

In the event of a widespread catastrophe, it's okay to look to the authorities for help and guidance, just don't take for granted that any assistance will be available. In other words, hope for the best, but plan for the worst. Assume that:

* Your normal energy sources, such as electricity, natural gas, gasoline, propane, etc., will be disabled.

* You will have no running water.

* You are not going to be rescued by the local fire department, paramedics, or any law enforcement agency.

* You are not going to get help from any public agencies such as the Federal Emergency Management Agency, the Centers for Disease Control, etc.

* You are not going to get help from any private agencies, such as the Red Cross.

Say that some event knocks out the power grid for an extended period. Without electricity, you don't have lights, and you don't have refrigeration. If it's summertime, you don't have air conditioning. If it's wintertime and you use electric heat, you don't have heat; even if you use gas heat, the electric blower won't work. If you have a well with an electric pump, you don't have water. You can't cook, you can't wash clothes, and you can't take a shower. Without electricity, grocery stores, pharmacies, and restaurants close. Traffic lights don't work. Gas pumps don't work. ATMs don't work. Schools close. Factories close. Offices close. When people don't work, they don't get paid, and then they can't pay their bills. The event cascades into a bigger and bigger problem.

If officials don't provide an adequate response to a disaster, be prepared to take action on your own. You don't always have to be an "expert" to know what to do. Use the knowledge and skills that you have gained to help yourself out of a bad situation.

Don't allow other people's inaction to influence you to do nothing. Sometimes people don't take action because of the "bystander effect," the tendency of people to stand by and do nothing as a catastrophic event unfolds. This may happen because as the number of bystanders increases, any given bystander is less likely to assume responsibility for taking action. Everyone assumes that someone else is going to take care of things. Don't hesitate to take action. Take the lead!

You can't control many of the events that happen to you, but you can control how you respond to them. Train yourself to be ready to handle whatever comes your way. Be proactive. Practice emergency drills. Live with confidence.

Crisis can bring out the best in people or the worst in people. Let it bring out the best in you.

I. M. Reddy

Contents

Contents

Contents

Contents

Contents

Contents

WHY PREPARE FOR DISASTERS

Reason #1: No one is immune from disaster; catastrophes can happen to anyone, regardless of income, geography, or other factors. Rich people who build multi-million dollar homes overlooking the beach are just as much at risk as poor people who live in trailer parks on the prairie.

Reason #2: The more prepared you are, the greater your chances of survival. The more serious a catastrophic event is, the more your preparedness will pay off.

Reason #3: It's better to have control over your own life than to leave it in the hands of other people. Like it or not, you depend heavily on others for your survival, and you need to reduce that dependence. For example, you depend on a farmer to grow your food, you depend on a migrant worker to harvest your food, you depend on a trucker to transport your food to a processing plant, you depend on a machine operator to process your food, you depend on another trucker to deliver your food to a grocery store, and you depend on a grocer to sell it to you. A dozen different things could go wrong, but look at what would happen if just one thing changed. It's easy to imagine the price of fuel skyrocketing. If that happens, the farmer may not be able to buy fuel for his tractor, the migrant worker may not be able to afford to travel from field to field, the truckers may not be able to buy fuel for their rigs, the machine operator may not be able to afford to commute to work, and so on. If any link in this supply chain is broken, you will be without food.

If you still need to be convinced on the idea of emergency preparedness, just turn on the evening news and listen to the recurring stories: terrorist bombings, chemical spills, explosions, blizzards, blackouts, fires, earthquakes, volcanoes, hurricanes, tornadoes, floods, financial collapse, civil unrest, and other calamities. It never ends.

Introduction

HOW TO USE THIS BOOK

This book is divided into three sections: Before, During, and After.

Section 1, "Before," is about minimizing damage and making preparations prior to a disaster. It includes chapters on:

- sheltering-in-place plans and evacuation plans
- communication plans
- how to mitigate property damage and personal injury
- supplies to stockpile
- tools and equipment to have
- personal habits that can help minimize your exposure to danger
- what to do beforehand to make recovery easier in the aftermath of a disaster
- how to prepare for an apocalyptic event that permanently changes your lifestyle
- maintaining your readiness once your plans are in place

At the end of each chapter, you'll find worksheets and checklists that summarize the tasks covered in that chapter. You'll also find lists of items to acquire. You may want to review these lists before you read each chapter, in conjunction with reading the text, or instead of reading the text. (Who doesn't like a shortcut? If you skip the text and go straight to the lists, you won't be alone!)

Section 2, "During," outlines what to do during different kinds of catastrophic events. Reading through this section before disaster strikes will help you know what to do when the time comes. It includes:

- general responses that apply to all emergencies
- responses that apply to specific kinds of emergencies, alphabetized to make it easy to find the material you need to refer to

Section 3, "After," outlines actions to take in the aftermath. It includes chapters on:

- how to get back to "normal" if recovery is possible
- how to adjust to a "new normal" if an apocalyptic event occurs

How well you prepare will depend on how much time and money you have to devote to the project, as well as your level of enthusiasm (or sense of urgency). Ultimately, how much preparation you do is up to you. You can stash a box of crackers and a jar of peanut butter in the back of the pantry and probably survive a power outage that lasts a couple of days. Take it to the next level and store several cases of water and dehydrated food and you'll probably survive many major disasters. Kick it up another notch and learn how to raise crops, slaughter livestock, and weave your own cloth. Or you can become a hardcore survivalist and learn how to live off the land with next to nothing, making you one of the few who will be able to survive a cataclysmic event such as a nuclear winter.

Whether you want to do a little or a lot of emergency preparedness, this book has something for everyone. You can devote a weekend to emergency preparedness, or you can make survivalism a lifestyle.

Some of the suggestions are habits that you can adopt right away, such as filling your vehicle with fuel whenever it reaches half a tank. Other suggestions are specific tasks to accomplish and may take weeks or even months to complete, such as repairing leaky faucets, reinforcing your roof, or changing your landscaping.

Some may be repetitive tasks, such as stockpiling supplies and rotating perishables, while other tasks may need to be performed only once and then updated on a regular basis, such as gathering and organizing documents.

Some suggestions don't require any money, such as keeping shoes by your bed for a quick escape. Others require a little money, such as buying a fireproof cabinet to store flammable liquids. And some require a substantial amount of money, such as installing a tornado shelter.

It's unlikely that you'll do everything this book suggests, but anything you do to prepare for emergencies is better than doing nothing at all. Even small steps can mean the difference between life and death.

Sometimes this book states the obvious, because in an emergency, people don't always think clearly. People in emergency situations often lose their heads and can't think logically about what to do, but they may remember something they've read.

Introduction

Practice, practice, practice. Practice your skills so you'll know what to do in any emergency. If you make your emergency response behavior become second nature, you won't freeze in the midst of an emergency, you won't be in denial, and you won't have to deliberate with yourself or others to decide what to do.

As you work through your emergency preparedness project, remember that the keys to survival are:

▶ **Attitude** - Have a positive attitude and develop a survivalist mindset. This doesn't mean to live like a hermit and greet everyone at your door with a shotgun. It does mean that you need to have a realistic understanding of what your risks are and to learn the skills required to cope with those risks. Be proactive rather than reactive. When things don't go as planned in your life, don't act like a helpless victim; instead, do what you can to take control of your situation. Keep things in perspective and be resilient. Believe that you can do what it takes to survive and thrive.

▶ **Resourcefulness and Adaptability** - Always think about how everyday items can be used in a different way. Use your imagination!

▶ **Redundancy** - Since you can't predict what kind of emergencies will occur and how they will disrupt your life, your chances of survival are highest if you give yourself multiple levels of protection. For example, electrical devices won't work if you lose electric power, but you could have a generator as a backup. However, your generator won't work if you run out of fuel for it, so you could also have solar-powered devices as backups. However, solar-powered devices won't work if the sun's rays are blocked by rain clouds or dust clouds, so you could also have manually operated devices as backups. In all aspects of emergency preparedness – food sources, tools, energy, etc. - give yourself as many options as possible.

Before Disaster

This section outlines ways you can prepare for an emergency before one happens. This section includes the following nine chapters:

Chapter 1 helps you develop **sheltering-in-place and evacuation plans** for your home, your vehicle, your workplace, and other locations. It helps you establish a budget, set priorities, and establish deadlines for achieving your goals.

Chapter 2 helps you develop a **communications plan**.

Chapter 3 outlines actions you can take to **mitigate property damage and personal injury.**

Chapter 4 lists expendable **supplies** that you need to have.

Chapter 5 lists durable **tools and equipment** that you need to have.

Chapter 6 outlines **personal practices** that can help you minimize your exposure to mishaps.

Chapter 7 helps you develop a plan for **recovery** and a return to "normal" after a disaster.

Chapter 8 helps you prepare for an **apocalypse** that permanently changes your lifestyle.

Chapter 9 outlines a **maintenance plan** for your readiness once you have your plans in place, you have fortified your dwelling, and you have a stockpile of supplies and equipment.

Chapter 1

Emergency Response Plans

In response to an emergency, you have two choices: shelter-in-place or evacuate. The response you choose will depend on the nature of the emergency and how well prepared you are.

One catastrophic event can lead to another, so it's best to prepare for more than one kind of catastrophe, taking into account the geography and other factors where you live. An earthquake can not only topple buildings, it can also rupture gas lines and cause fires. An earthquake can trigger a tsunami that in turn can trigger a nuclear meltdown (Japan, 2011). An earthquake can also trigger a volcanic eruption; likewise, a volcanic eruption can trigger an earthquake, as well as other catastrophic events, such as severe thunderstorms, flash floods, and landslides. A hurricane nearly always leads to flooding; after Katrina in 2005, the city of New Orleans went from bad to worse as it descended into looting and civil unrest. A hurricane can also spawn tornadoes farther inland. A heat wave may lead to a drought that in turn may lead to wildfires or dust storms (Texas, 2011).

Be willing to adapt to your circumstances. Always have a backup plan. If Plan A doesn't work, be prepared to go to Plan B; if Plan B doesn't work, be prepared to go to Plan C.

The topics in this chapter include:

- sheltering-in-place and evacuation
- outlining your plans
- budget
- priorities
- deadlines

SHELTER-IN-PLACE

Shelter-in-place means to take cover wherever you are: at home, at work, at school, in your vehicle, in a public building downtown, or inside a cave in the woods. It is intended to be "temporary," but that's a relative term. Temporary may mean a few minutes for an event such as riding out an earthquake or waiting for a thunderstorm to pass. It may mean a few hours for an event such as a power outage. It may mean several days for an event such as enduring a blizzard. In extreme cases, you may need to shelter-in-place for an extended period of time, from a couple of weeks to a couple of months, for events such as a nuclear attack or a pandemic.

Be prepared to shelter-in-place anywhere you may be caught in an emergency. Develop shelter-in-place plans for:

- ◆ your home
- ◆ your vehicles
- ◆ your workplace or an urban public place
- ◆ a rural or wilderness setting

EVACUATE

Evacuate means to leave your current location and move to a safer place, but that can mean many different things. It may mean moving a short distance, such as getting outside of a burning building, or it may mean moving a long distance, such as traveling several miles to get away from the effects of a chemical spill. If you have to evacuate your building at work, you may simply be able to go home, depending on the nature of the disaster and how widespread it is. If you have to evacuate your home, you may go to a public shelter, a hotel, a relative's house in another city, or some other facility.

Evacuation is usually temporary, such as to escape a flood, but in extreme cases, it may be permanent, for events such as a landslide that permanently wipes your property off the map.

Develop evacuation plans for:

♦   a temporary situation, when return and recovery are likely
♦   a permanent situation, when return and recovery are unlikely

OUTLINE YOUR EMERGENCY RESPONSE PLANS

Think not only about the kinds of disasters you might face in your own environment, but also about how disasters in other places can affect you, sometimes for a long period of time. For instance, if you live in the Great Plains, a hurricane probably isn't going to destroy your home, but if a hurricane destroys an oil refinery on the Gulf coast, everyone is going to experience fuel shortages and price increases in fuel, including those living as far away as the Great Plains. Fuel shortages lead in turn to food shortages and price increases in food as well.

Anything that affects the availability and price of one commodity usually has a ripple effect on the availability and prices of other commodities. Maybe you like shellfish, but you don't eat much shrimp, so you think any disaster that hits the shrimping industry won't affect your food budget. However, people who do eat shrimp and can no longer get it are going to look for substitutes to satisfy their seafood habit. So they start eating more clams, crabs, and lobster. If the demand for these other shellfish goes up, but the supply doesn't, the prices will go up as well. So you and millions of other people switch to chicken, and then the price of chicken goes up!

The point is, we live in a complex, global economy. Events that seem small or remote can have wide-ranging effects. It's the "butterfly effect:" a seemingly insignificant event at one time and place can result in significant events at another time and place.

Also consider what emergencies might come up when you travel, either for business or for pleasure. You might be in an unfamiliar climate and in unfamiliar terrain. Consider how you would deal with strange surroundings and unknown resources. If you travel internationally, you might also encounter a language barrier.

❑ Identify who is included in your group.

♦ How many people and animals live in your household? How many others are dependent on you now, or will be in the future? Will you be having more children, or do you have grown children who will be leaving the nest? Will you have elderly parents moving in with you, or moving out to a nursing home?

♦ What are the needs of your group members? Does your group include babies, small children, the elderly, the disabled, or someone with a chronic medical condition? Do you need to stockpile diapers and formula, oxygen tanks, syringes, or other medical equipment and supplies?

♦ What are the abilities of your group members? Can they dress and feed themselves? Can they be left alone, or do they require supervision? How much weight can they lift? What tools are they capable of using?

♦ If you share custody of children, think about your plan of action if a catastrophic event happens while the children are with the other parent.

♦ If you have students away at school, think about the arrangements you need to make for contacting or meeting them.

♦ If you have elderly parents who live on their own, think about which sibling will have primary responsibility for their welfare in an emergency.

♦ If you have elderly parents in a nursing home, consider under what circumstances you would remove them from the facility and keep them with your immediate family.

♦ If you travel for work, consider alternate means of transportation and alternate routes that you might have to use to return home.

♦ If you are a business owner, think about the arrangements you need to make to protect your employees and your livelihood.

♦ What special circumstances apply to your group?

Before Disaster

❑ Assign tasks to appropriate members of your group:

    ❑ Upgrade your dwelling.

    ❑ Purchase, organize, and rotate supplies.

    ❑ Purchase and maintain equipment and tools.

    ❑ Take photos of your assets and maintain electronic files and hard copies of important documents.

    ❑ Safeguard cash.

    ❑ Pick up the children at school in case of an emergency.

    ❑ Communicate with your long-distance contacts when an emergency arises.

❑ Decide where you will meet.

    ❑ In case of an emergency inside your home, designate a place to meet right outside your home so all family members and pets can be accounted for quickly.

    ❑ In case of an emergency away from home, designate a place to meet. If a disaster happens during the day when family members are scattered at school, work, and other places, think about the best place to meet. Most of your sheltering-in-place and evacuation supplies will be stored at home, so meeting at home is generally the first choice; then you can shelter-in-place together at home or evacuate together. However, if authorities direct you to shelter-in-place wherever you are, you will have to wait until it is safe to travel before returning home, or if it isn't safe to return home, you must have an alternate meeting place outside of your neighborhood. Also think about how members of the group will be able to communicate among themselves about where they are.

❏ Think about whether you will shelter-in-place or evacuate.

Debate scenarios in which you would plan to shelter-in-place and those in which you would plan to evacuate. What conditions will determine whether to shelter-in-place or evacuate, i.e., what is your threshold for each kind of emergency situation? Is it when the floodwaters are lapping at your front door? Is it when a wildfire is half a mile away?

In planning your disaster responses, take your habitat into account. Consider not only where you live now, but where you might relocate in case of an evacuation. For example, to stay in or evacuate to a cold climate, you need warm clothing. Near water, you may need boating and fishing gear.

Consider whether all members of your group are capable of walking a significant distance, if escaping on foot is the only means out.

Maybe you don't want to stockpile supplies, so your plan is always to evacuate. But what would you do if you are quarantined?

When an emergency arises, the decision to stay or go may be clear. If you're unsure, you'll have to assess the situation at the time, but you should already have the pro's and con's summarized in your mind so you can make a decision quickly. Be prepared to make the decision that will save your life.

The timescale of an event can vary from a few seconds (an explosion) to a few minutes (an earthquake) to a few hours (a hurricane) to days (a volcanic eruption) and even to years (a drought) or decades (nuclear contamination). You must be prepared to act immediately, as soon as an incident occurs, and to continue dealing with the crisis during its acute phase and through its chronic aftermath.

❏ Learn the locations of all clinics and hospitals in your vicinity, as well as some outside your area.

During a widespread catastrophic event, emergency facilities will become overcrowded, and you may have to travel beyond the closest one to receive treatment.

SHELTER-IN-PLACE AT HOME

☐ Be prepared with:
- ◆ supplies to seal off your safe room or entire home
- ◆ emergency lighting
- ◆ alternate heat source and/or blankets
- ◆ emergency power for appliances: batteries or generator
- ◆ communications equipment: radio, phone, computer, etc.
- ◆ prescription medications
- ◆ bottled water
- ◆ food supplies that don't require refrigeration or cooking
- ◆ sanitation supplies such as soap and bleach
- ◆ snow removal equipment: shovel, blower, tractor blade, de-icing salt or other chemicals, etc.
- ◆ books, board games, playing cards, arts and crafts, etc.

For any emergency when water may be in short supply, be prepared to draw water into every available fixture to supplement the water you will already have in storage.

☐ Assign at least one person to the task of filling up the kitchen sink, bathroom sinks, bathtubs, utility sink, clothes washer, and any other available container with water.

In the event of a biological, chemical, or nuclear accident or attack, you will need to turn off all ventilation systems and seal your windows and other openings with plastic and duct tape. (More on this topic in the chapter entitled "Mitigate Property Damage & Personal Injury." For now, think about who is capable of performing these tasks.)

☐ Assign a member of your group to be responsible for turning off ventilation systems in your shelter.

☐ Assign a team of two people to be responsible for sealing openings of your shelter.

☐ Assign a member of your group to be responsible for stripping and decontaminating children before entering your shelter.

☐ Assign a member of your group to be responsible for decontaminating animals and herding them inside.

SHELTER-IN-PLACE IN YOUR VEHICLE

Typical scenarios in which you might have to stay in your vehicle would be if you were caught in a snowstorm, if a rockslide blocks the road, if a flood knocks out a bridge, if an earthquake buckles the pavement, or some other event prevents your movement.

❏ Keep each vehicle's fuel tank full and keep each vehicle stocked with:
  ◆ supplies to seal off vents
  ◆ flashlight or lantern
  ◆ warm clothing or blankets
  ◆ bottled water
  ◆ food snacks that don't require refrigeration or cooking
  ◆ sanitation supplies such as disposable wipes
  ◆ shovel with sand or kitty litter
  ◆ tire chains
  ◆ goggles
  ◆ masks
  ◆ petroleum jelly to apply to the insides of your nostrils to keep them from drying out during a dust storm

SHELTER-IN-PLACE IN AN URBAN PUBLIC SETTING

An emergency may happen when you're at your job, out shopping, at a concert, working out at the gym, attending a sporting event, or dong any one of a hundred other things.

Your employer may have plans to safeguard you and your co-workers for a short period of time until imminent danger passes. Government agencies and large employers have disaster plans, but many small businesses do not. (You know your bosses; can you count on them?) If you work for a small business, be prepared to take care of yourself. If possible, store some nonperishable food and bottled water in your desk, locker, or other personal space. During a crisis, you may not have access to the supplies in your vehicle.

It's impractical to carry around blankets and a case of bottled water wherever you go, so any emergency that happens when you are out in public is going to catch you without a lot of survival supplies. However, you can carry a few basic items in a handbag, fanny pack, backpack, or briefcase. These items constitute your "get-home bag." They can also serve as sheltering-in-place supplies if you are forced to seek shelter while away from home.

❑ Keep these critical items with you:
- prescription medications (three-day supply)
- bottled water
- food snacks that don't require refrigeration or cooking
- sanitation supplies such as a small bottle of hand sanitizer or prepackaged wet wipes
- mask
- foam ear plugs
- bandana in a bright color such as red, yellow, or orange
- miniature flashlight
- small pry bar
- window punch
- comfortable walking shoes

SHELTER-IN-PLACE IN A RURAL OR WILDERNESS AREA

You may become stranded in a rural area while camping or hiking, in which case you may have some basic necessities with you. Or you may become stranded while driving through a remote area, in which case you may have some supplies in your vehicle. Surviving in the wilderness means using whatever is available to you. Learn basic survival skills:

- how to build a temporary shelter

- how to build a fire

- how to find and purify water

- how to find food

- how to communicate with rescuers

These are the same skills you will need for your apocalypse plan. For more information on developing these skills, see the chapter entitled "Apocalypse Plan."

EVACUATE FROM DWELLING

❑ Draw the floor plan of your dwelling and mark two escape routes out of each bedroom and living space. Make sure your children understand the routes.

❑ Keep exit routes clear.

❑ Keep a loud bell and a flashlight next to each bed. If evacuation is necessary, you will ring the bell to alert other members of the household, and use the flashlight to find your way out.

❑ Keep slip-on shoes or slippers by each bedside in case you need to leave the house quickly due to a fire, flash flood, earthquake, or other sudden event.

❑ Store collapsible ladders in all bedrooms that are above the ground floor.

❑ Install fire extinguishers in the kitchen and near other sources of potential fire hazards, such as a fireplace, space heaters, etc.

❑ Locate the utility shutoffs for electricity, gas, and water. Every adult member of your group should know where they are located and how to turn them off. (The gas valve is closed when the tang [the part you put the wrench on] is crosswise of the pipe.) Note that if you shut off the gas, only a representative from the gas company can turn it back on. You will have to wait until a technician is available to perform this service for you, and you will probably have to pay a fee for this service, so only turn off the gas if safety warrants it.

❑ Designate a place to meet right outside your home so all family members and pets can be accounted for quickly.

❑ Identify the closest higher ground and determine how you would reach it in the event of a flash flood.

EVACUATE FROM WORKPLACE

❑ Learn where fire extinguishers are located, and be sure you know how to use them.

❑ Familiarize yourself with the facility's layout. Establish a primary escape route as well as an alternate escape route.

❑ Know the "landmarks" along your escape route. Count the number of desks or cubicles or doors between your workspace and the closest exit so you can find your way even in thick smoke or complete darkness.

❑ Find out where to report for roll call and to whom. Your employer should designate an assembly area away from the building, and appoint someone to take a head count for each department, so that all employees can be accounted for in case the building must be evacuated. Appropriate places to take refuge would be an adjacent parking lot, a nearby sidewalk, or an open field.

TEMPORARY EVACUATION

A voluntary evacuation order means you are advised to leave the area but are not required to do so. The advantage to leaving early is that you may get out ahead of the congestion on the evacuation routes.

A mandatory evacuation means that only emergency personnel are authorized to remain in the area. If you stay, you won't be arrested, but you won't be rescued, either.

❑ Learn about your community's emergency evacuation plan.

❑ Familiarize yourself with the emergency plans of your employer, your children's day care center and schools, the nursing facility of a disabled or elderly family member, etc. Find out where your children or other relatives would be taken if their facility is evacuated.

❑ Learn the location of public emergency shelters in your area. Teach your children to recognize signs for "Safe Place," "Emergency Shelter," "Tornado Shelter," "Fallout Shelter," "Evacuation Route," and other emergency signage in your area. Make sure all family members know how to reach them from home, school, and work.

Public shelters provide just that: shelter. They are not resorts. Ordinarily, they do not provide food, water, sanitation, bedding, or medical care. If a crisis is expected to last more than a few hours, other agencies may step in and provide those support services, but it may take some time for them to respond.

❑ Make a list of places you can go to get relief from heat, such as a shopping mall, a theater, a library, a pool or water park, etc. Your community may also have "cooling centers" where you can go to escape the heat.

❑ Consider where else you could go in an emergency:
   ♦ a weekend or vacation home
   ♦ friends or relatives in another area who can take you in
   ♦ hotel

❑ Become familiar with various means of public transportation out of your area, such as buses or trains. In the event of a disaster, mass transportation will quickly become overwhelmed, but if you leave early, you may beat the rush.

❑ Drive the evacuation routes out of your area and determine what your proposed destination would be in each direction. Every family member should know the main evacuation routes as well as alternate routes.

❑ Think about alternatives to driving a car or walking: rollerblades, ice skates, snow skis, snowmobiles, dogsleds, horses, bicycles, motorcycles, and various kinds of watercraft.

❑ If you live in a large city, public transportation is likely to be overcrowded and may even be out of service because of the emergency. Likewise, the roadways are likely to become impassable as they become choked with vehicles. Consider how this might affect the timing of your decision to evacuate.

❑ Think about what you will take with you.
  ◆ Prescription medications, water, and food should be top priorities.
  ◆ For clothing, consider the climate you would likely be exposed to.
  ◆ Consider how long you expect to be away.
  ◆ Consider how much space you have in the mode of transportation that is likely to be available to you.
  ◆ If you are planning to stay with friends or relatives far removed from the disaster, you may need to take very little with you.
  ◆ If you plan to stay in a hotel and you have plenty of money for living expenses, you may need to take very little with you.
  ◆ Remember that everyday stuff can be replaced. Other than life-supporting necessities, only small items that have a great deal of sentimental value and are truly irreplaceable should be taken with you.
  ◆ Whatever containers you use -- plastic bins, boxes, luggage, backpacks, duffel bags – be sure family members are able to carry them.

PERMANENT EVACUATION

The landscape may be altered permanently by floodwaters, mudslides, lava flows or other conditions to the extent that you really can't go home again.

❑ Your first priority, as always, is to save yourself and your loved ones. Be prepared to take whatever you need to survive.

❑ After the critical life-sustaining stuff, make room for some items that have sentimental value and are truly irreplaceable, such as photos or small family keepsakes.

❑ Your everyday stuff can be replaced and most of it may be covered by insurance. Be prepared to let it go.

BUDGET

Create a budget for your survival needs. Consider how much money you are willing to spend now and in the future and divide your budget among the various categories where you need to upgrade your readiness, such as dwelling improvements, supplies, and equipment. Water, life-sustaining medications, and food should be high on your list of supplies.

You have several ways to fund your survival purchases:

- ♦ **Convert existing assets.** Use cash out of savings or sell items by having a garage sale, using a consignment shop, marketing through an online auction, etc.

- ♦ **Decrease expenses.** Reduce what you spend on other goods and services and reallocate the difference to your survival budget. (Change your insurance deductibles, eat in instead of out, rent a movie instead of buying theater tickets, etc.)

- ♦ **Increase income.** Work overtime or take on a second job for extra money.

Think of survival planning as an insurance policy, but instead of paying someone else to insure you against losses, you're spending the money to buy the supplies and equipment you need to protect yourself.

If you can't afford to spend much money on this project, start with the things that are free. For example, it doesn't cost anything for you to learn where "Safe Place" and "Fallout Shelter" signs are located in your community. Then move on to the things that are very low cost, such as storing tap water in recycled juice bottles. You may not be as well prepared for a disaster as you could be if you had more money, but anything you do to prepare is better than doing nothing at all.

PRIORITIES

Review the disasters that you are most likely to encounter to determine which purchases are most important to you. For example, if you live in Kansas, having a tornado shelter is a high priority for you. If you live in California, your time and money are best spent preparing for the next earthquake.

Your personal safety is more important than protecting your possessions, so actions you can take to safeguard yourself and your loved ones are obviously a higher priority than safeguarding your property. However, many tactics for protecting your house can also improve your personal safety if you are sheltering-in-place at home during a disaster, so such mitigation techniques can serve dual purposes.

DEADLINES

Break this project into small manageable tasks, and set realistic target dates for accumulating the cash you need, purchasing supplies and equipment, retrofitting your home, and learning and practicing survival skills.

Start buying extra food supplies on a weekly or monthly basis. Add these items to your regular grocery-shopping trip, or set aside one night of the week to visit a sporting goods store to acquire the supplies and equipment you need, or devote one Saturday a month to the project. Do whatever works for you. Once you reach a minimum level for survival, start rotating your stock and replace older items with newer ones.

As funds allow, start buying other items such as first aid supplies, paper goods, tools, equipment, etc., as well as home improvements such as a safe room, storm shutters, rain barrels, etc., and take training classes to learn survival skills.

Response Plans

Who is included in our group (people and animals): _____

_____

_____

Special needs we have: _____

_____

Capabilities and limitations of our group members: _____

_____

_____

Where our supplies are stored: _____

_____

Who is responsible for picking up children: _____

_____

Names and addresses of nearest hospitals:

_____

_____

_____

_____

Sheltering-In-Place At Home

Who is responsible for securing shelter:

Strip and decontaminate children before entering shelter. _____

_____

_____

Decontaminate animals and herd them inside. _____

_____

_____

Turn off ventilation systems. _____

_____

Seal openings. _____

_____

Draw water. _____

_____

Unlock weapons and ammunition. _____

_____

Communicate with long-distance contact. _____

_____

Evacuation

Where we will meet if evacuating home: _____

_____

Where we will meet if evacuating out of area: _____

_____

Alternate meeting place: _____

_____

Who is responsible for shutting off utilities: _____

_____

Names and addresses of nearest emergency shelters:

_____

_____

_____

_____

_____

Budget

_____	Water
_____	Food
_____	Medications & Medical Supplies
_____	Sanitation Supplies
_____	Clothing, Bedding, Masks, Filters
_____	Cash
_____	Pet Supplies
_____	Power-generating Supplies & Equipment
_____	Communications Equipment
_____	Other Tools & Equipment
_____	Vehicles
_____	Library
_____	Insurance
_____	Weapons & Ammunition
_____	Dwelling Interior
_____	Dwelling Exterior
_____	Landscape
_____	Other_____
_____	Other_____
_____	Other_____

Priorities

_____

_____

_____

_____

_____

_____

_____

_____

_____

_____

_____

_____

_____

_____

_____

_____

Deadlines

_____

_____

_____

_____

_____

_____

_____

_____

_____

_____

_____

_____

_____

_____

_____

_____

Chapter 2

Communications Plan

This chapter discusses the actions to take to develop a communications plan so your group members can reach one another during a crisis. For a list of communications equipment to help you implement your plan, refer to the chapter entitled "Tools & Equipment."

❑ Memorize the names, addresses, and phone numbers of emergency contacts. Don't rely on your cell phone; if the battery runs out, you won't have access to your contact list.

❑ Obtain other useful emergency phone numbers and keep them handy. Store them in your cell phone contact list, and keep a written list near your land line at home. Examples: hospital, fire and rescue, poison control center, etc. These numbers could be invaluable if your local 911 call center were to become jammed during an emergency.

❑ Every cell phone contact list should have an entry for "ICE" that stands for "In Case of Emergency" and stores the name and number of the person to be notified. Emergency personnel are trained to look for this entry when dealing with an incapacitated individual. If you have more than one, use ICE 1 as your primary emergency contact, ICE 2 as your secondary emergency contact, and so on.

❑ Establish a communication chain. Decide in advance who is responsible for contacting other group members at the onset of an emergency.

❑ Designate an out-of-state relative or friend as an emergency contact. If you have problems communicating with members of your group through local channels, you may be able to relay information through your long-distance contact. Have both a primary and a secondary long-distance contact.

❑ Have an emergency code word shared by all members of your group. This word is used to set your emergency plan in motion. If you receive a phone call, voicemail, text message, email, or any other communication from a group member with this word, you should proceed to your predetermined meeting place.

❑ Have one central location in your home for group members to check for messages. It can be a corkboard, a blackboard, a whiteboard, or a piece of paper stuck to the refrigerator with a magnet. In the event of an evacuation, if group members arrive home at different times, they can look at the message board to find out which other members have checked in and who has proceeded to the designated meeting spot.

❑ Be sure all members of your group know how to use the resources that may be available in an emergency.

    ❑ Teach all members to tune in to a radio or TV station to listen to the Emergency Alert System. During an emergency, this network disseminates information and updates on how a disaster is unfolding, including areas affected, the expected duration of the event, and other information from authorities.

    ❑ Become familiar with the sound of your community's warning siren or other alarm system.

    ❑ Teach your children how to reverse phone charges so they can make a call from a public phone without change in an emergency.

    ❑ Teach your children how to contact you via email.

❑ Give your children a secret password that no one would be able to guess, and teach them to require this password from any stranger who approaches them and claims to have instructions from you about what to do in an unfamiliar situation. Make sure your children understand the difference between following the instructions of a police officer or firefighter who is a stranger, versus following the instructions of a stranger who wants your child to "help look for a lost puppy."

Communications Plan

❏ Memorize the names, addresses, and phone numbers of emergency contacts.

❏ Obtain other useful emergency phone numbers. Store them in your cell phone contact list and keep a written list near your land line at home.

❏ Set up "ICE" entries in your cell phone contact list to store the name and number of the person to be notified in case of emergency.

❏ Establish a communication chain.

❏ Designate out-of-state relatives or friends as emergency contacts.

❏ Have an emergency code word, shared by all members of your group, to set your emergency plan in motion.

❏ Have one central location in your home for group members to check for messages.

❏ Be sure all members of your group know how to use the resources that may be available in an emergency.

    ❏ Teach all members to tune in to a radio or TV station to listen to the Emergency Alert System.

    ❏ Become familiar with the sound of your community's warning siren or other alarm system.

    ❏ Teach your children how to reverse phone charges.

    ❏ Teach your children how to contact you via email.

❏ Give your children a secret password and teach them to require this password from strangers who approach them.

Phone Numbers

Home... _____
Cell.. _____
Cell.. _____
Cell.. _____
Cell.. _____
Work... _____
Work... _____
Work... _____
Work... _____
Daycare.. _____
School.. _____
School.. _____
Police... _____
Sheriff.. _____
State Patrol.. _____
Road Conditions... _____
Fire Department... _____
Doctor.. _____
Doctor.. _____
Doctor.. _____
Hospital.. _____
Hospital.. _____
Hospital.. _____
Vet... _____
Animal Hospital.. _____
Electric Utility.. _____
Gas Utility... _____
Water Utility... _____
Phone Company... _____
Internet Service Provider............................. _____
Cable/Satellite Dish Service Provider............ _____
Alarm Service.. _____
Medical Alert Service................................... _____
Poison Control.. 800-222-1222
CDC Chemical/Biological/Radiological Hotline................. 888-246-2675
CDC Immunization Hotline.. 800-232-2522
State Emergency Management Agency........... _____
Federal Emergency Management Agency...................... 800-621-3362
State Environmental Protection Agency............ _____
Federal Environmental Protection Agency...................... 800-424-8802
_____....... _____

Chapter 3

Mitigate Property Damage & Personal Injury

This chapter discusses actions you can take inside and outside your home to lessen the impact of disasters. A property mitigation plan involves taking steps to minimize damage to your real property (your house and the land it sits on) and your personal property (your big-screen TV and computer, your furniture, and those precious family heirlooms you inherited from your in-laws). If you are forced to shelter in place at home, many of the steps you take to mitigate property damage will mitigate personal injury as well.

Some changes can be made quickly and inexpensively. Others will require more time, effort, expense, and in some cases, professional help. Your money will be well spent, since it's usually cheaper to prevent damage than to repair it.

For the latest mitigation techniques in new construction, consult with professionals: an architect regarding building construction, a civil engineer regarding the underlying soil, and a landscaper regarding vegetation.

You can also retrofit existing construction. Complex projects will undoubtedly require you to hire an experienced contractor, but some of the easier projects are well within the capabilities of the average do-it-yourselfer; just strap on your tool belt and go for it!

If your home was built before the current building codes were established, you may need to consult an engineer or architect about securing and reinforcing your home's foundation, walls, floor joists, roof joists, and chimneys.

Understand your risks. Learn from the past and assess what you need to do to mitigate damage. Become informed about your area's potential for various disasters and what resources are available to you. Consider not just the statistical probability that a certain catastrophe will occur, but what will happen to you if it does.

The topics in this chapter include:

- dwelling interior
- dwelling exterior
- landscaping

DWELLING INTERIOR

Loose Objects

Securing loose objects not only helps prevent damage to your possessions, but also helps prevent them from hurting you by falling on you or becoming projectiles during an earthquake, high winds, or other powerful event.

❑ Strap your water heater to wall studs.

❑ If you have a free-standing stove, bolt it to the floor or the wall.

❑ Ensure that light fixtures and ceiling fans are hung securely.

❑ Move pictures, mirrors, and other wall-hangings away from beds.

❑ Bolt shelves and other furniture to wall studs to keep them from toppling over.

❑ Add molding to the edges of open shelves to create lips to keep objects from sliding off.

❑ Anchor objects to shelves or tables with adhesive or putty.

❑ Install latches on cabinet doors to keep them closed.

❑ Secure electronics such as TV's and computers.

❑ Store hazardous materials such as gasoline, cleaners, fertilizers, and other chemicals in approved containers. Place the containers in sturdy fire-resistant cabinets bolted to the wall or place them on the floor of the garage or storage shed rather than on open shelves.

To avoid confusion:
- ◆ Gasoline is usually stored in a red container.
- ◆ Diesel is usually stored in a yellow container.
- ◆ Kerosene is usually stored in a blue container.
- ◆ Two-stroke fuel is usually stored in a green container.

Interior Window Coverings

❏ Install insulated draperies, shades, or blinds on your windows to keep the hot sun from shining into your home during a heat wave.

❏ Be prepared to cover all exterior openings of your shelter on the inside with plastic sheeting to protect yourself from biological toxins, volcanic ash, or other airborne contaminants.

◆ Have enough plastic sheeting and duct tape to cover all exterior doors, windows, and vents. Measure the square footage of each opening to determine how much plastic sheeting to buy, and measure the perimeter of each opening to determine how much duct tape to buy.

◆ Use sheeting that is wide enough to cover the openings without creating seams.

◆ Use sheeting that is two to four milliliters thick.

◆ Cut the sheeting into pieces several inches larger than the openings and label each piece ("front door," "large bedroom window," etc.) in advance to save time in an emergency.

◆ Store the plastic covers with rolls of duct tape in a closet, cabinet, or other convenient place in each room so they will be readily accessible in an emergency.

Energy Usage

❏ Make sure your house is properly insulated. Install insulation in the attic and garage, and weather-stripping and caulking around exterior doors, windows, and vents. To determine if a window is leaking hot or cold air, hold a lighted candle next to the inside of the window, while someone else goes outside with a hair dryer and blows air along the frame. If the flame flickers, the window needs to be caulked.

❏ Make sure the seals are tight on the refrigerator and freezer. Replace them if necessary.

Filters

❑ Install HEPA filters. HEPA (High Efficiency Particle Arresting) filters are designed to remove airborne radioactive particles and many biological agents, as well as dust, dust mites, mold spores, pet dander, and allergens. HEPA filters are available for ventilation systems and vacuum cleaners.

Electrical

❑ Install smoke detectors in each bedroom and each living space.

❑ If you plan to use a portable generator during power outages, install an interlock or transfer switch on your home's electrical panel to make it safe and easy to convert your power source to your generator.

Plumbing

❑ Insulate your pipes to keep them from freezing during a power outage in cold weather.

❑ To minimize damage from earthquakes, use flexible tubing to connect gas appliances to rigid supply lines.

To minimize damage from flooding:

❑ Install backflow valves on all drains to prevent backups into your home.

❑ Install a sump pump with a battery backup; keep a spare on the shelf.

❑ Keep a gas-powered pump on site, along with fuel to operate it.

Reduce water consumption to fend off a water shortage:

❑ Repair leaky faucets.

❑ Attach flow restrictors or aerators to all sink faucets; install a low-flow shower head.

❑ Use a high-efficiency water-saving clothes washer and dishwasher.

Safe Room

To shelter-in-place during an intense event such as a tornado, you will need a "safe room," a part of your dwelling that you occupy to ride out the most severe conditions. Also known as a "survival room" or "panic room," it is a temporary containment shelter that can protect you from various threats. It can be designed to protect you from high winds, radiation, armed intruders, or other dangers.

If you are building a new home, consult your builder about including such a space in your new structure. Options may include pouring extra-thick concrete walls reinforced with rebar for your basement, lining your basement walls or a special room above ground with lead, or installing an above-ground or below-ground prefabricated steel vault. For existing homes, you can retrofit a space to serve as a safe room.

- It must be easy to seal off in case of a biological, chemical, or radiological disaster, so it should have no air conditioning, windows, doors, or vents to the outside. If it has exterior openings, be prepared to seal them with plastic and tape.

- The room should have a reinforced opening with a metal pocket door that slides from inside the adjoining wall, with a heavy-duty locking mechanism that is controlled from inside the room only. Having no knob or handle on the outside of the door offers the greatest protection from intruders.

- A room with only one opening means you may become trapped, but a single opening is easier to defend against intruders. A room with two openings is more difficult to defend, but offers a way to escape if one exit is blocked.

This room is where you should store your "core" emergency kit. Ideally, you will store all or most of your emergency supplies and equipment in your safe room, but due to space constraints, you may have to scatter your supplies and equipment throughout your dwelling. If this is the case, store the minimum that you need to survive for two or three days in the safe room, and retrieve extra supplies from other storage locations if the emergency lasts longer than that.

Mitigate Property Damage & Personal Injury

Include the following in your "core" emergency kit:

◆ water

◆ life-sustaining medications

◆ first-aid kit

◆ food

◆ sleeping bags or blankets and pillows

◆ bucket with lid and sanitation supplies if no flush toilet is in the room

◆ portable lighting, battery-powered or hand-cranked in case of a power outage

◆ radio or TV to listen for updates, battery-powered or hand-cranked in case of a power outage

◆ phone, a land line and/or a cell phone and its charger

◆ fire extinguisher

◆ folding escape ladder, if the room is located above the ground floor

◆ air horn, to discourage intruders or to alert rescue workers of your location

◆ strobe lights, to discourage intruders or to alert rescue workers of your location

◆ weapons and ammunition for group members old enough to shoot

DWELLING EXTERIOR

❑ Store bicycles and other loose items in the garage or a locked shed.

❑ If you have an LP gas tank on your property, secure it against high winds and earthquake tremors.

❑ If your structure is near water, keep sandbags, sand, and shovels ready to go in case the water rises.

❑ Install fire extinguishers outside near sources of fire, such as an outdoor fireplace, fire pit, or grill.

❑ Keep a can of International Orange spray paint on hand. If you have to evacuate your home during a widespread emergency, you will use it to mark your house to let rescuers know that it is unoccupied. Otherwise, they will break in to check for survivors.

Security

❑ Make sure your property is well lit on the outside to discourage criminals.

❑ Cut away dense undergrowth that could provide cover for an intruder.

❑ Erect a fence along the perimeter of your home or compound. Use barbed wire or razor wire for added security. If you electrify the fence, it can only be at a non-lethal voltage, and a minimum number of warning signs must be posted at eye level; it may also need to be installed within another, non-electrified, fence. Regardless of what kind of fence you erect, check with local authorities regarding building codes and permits required.

❑ Set trip wires that will activate an alarm if anyone breaches the perimeter of your property.

❑ Install solar-powered motion sensors with lights along your property lines and near your dwelling. Buy the highest wattage available. Position the lights to shine toward your dwelling when they come on, and position the light beams to intersect so you don't have areas hidden in darkness when the lights come on.

❑ Install surveillance cameras along your property lines and near your dwelling. Position them to capture activity from every angle leading to your dwelling, and hang them at an angle to get clear views of faces. Wire the cameras into a recording device.

❑ Install an alarm system with a loud horn on your dwelling. Install sensors on all doors and windows and wire them into the system.

❑ Get watch dogs and attack dogs. Watch dogs bark to warn you of strangers. Attack dogs assault strangers. Train them to keep them under your control.

❑ Never "hide" a key outside. Burglars know where to look.

Doors

❑ Install deadbolt locks on all exterior doors. Keep doors locked, even when you're at home.

❑ Install security gates on doorways to increase your protection against both crime and civil unrest.

❑ Reinforce entry doors and garage doors to keep out projectiles during hurricanes or tornadoes. Breached openings – broken doors and windows - cause air pressure to rise inside the structure, increasing the likelihood that the roof of the structure will be blown off. That's why it's important to do as much as possible to protect your doors and windows from being broken by flying debris during high winds.

Windows

❑ Install awnings over windows that receive direct sun to help keep your house cool and reduce energy usage.

❑ Install dual-pane or triple-pane windows. These reduce heat transfer, keeping your house warmer in winter and cooler in summer.

❑ To reduce breakability, install laminated glass or apply protective film to standard glass panes. It won't always keep glass from breaking, but if the glass does break, it will keep glass shards from scattering. It offers some resistance to forced entry, as well as some protection against earthquake tremors, flying debris in a tornado or hurricane, and the high heat of a fire. It can also reduce the heat of the sun coming in through the windows to help keep your house cool during a heat wave.

❑ Install steel bars or alarm mesh screens over windows. (Security bars have quick-release devices so you can still use the windows as emergency exits.)

❑ Purchase or fabricate shutters or other temporary covers to fit over doors, windows, vents, and any other openings of your structures. Drill holes in the middle of boards to equalize the pressure during a storm. Pre-drill holes and install anchors for nails or screws, depending on the material your shutter will be attached to. Label the boards so you'll be able to match each shutter to its opening in a hurry. Store the boards and installation hardware in a location that is easy to access in an emergency. These shutters can help diminish wind and water damage from a hurricane, can help reduce damage from a wildfire, and can help protect against breakage during civil unrest.

Roof & Gutters

The construction of your roof depends on factors such as climate, local building codes, availability of various materials, aesthetic design, and budget. Your roof can be made of any one of several different materials, such as metal, tile, stone, slate, shakes, wooden shingles, asphalt shingles, membranes of tar and rubber, or some other material.

Metal roofs are durable and long-lasting. They offer excellent protection against hail, wind, and fire. Depending on their finish, they can be very energy-efficient. They are low-maintenance and recyclable. They are also expensive.

Roofs made of tile, stone, or slate are also durable and long-lasting. The materials themselves offer excellent protection against hail, wind, and fire, but they must have special anchoring systems to be effective. Because of their weight, they must have adequate support. They are also relatively expensive.

Shakes, wooden shingles, and asphalt shingles can offer sufficient protection against the elements, but they must be properly secured to be effective.

❑ Use materials that are resistant to hail, wind, fire, and earthquakes, as well as energy-efficient:

- ◆ For the greatest fire resistance, use Class A fire-rated roofing materials.

- ◆ If you are using shingles, use wind-resistant shingles that are less likely to be pulled off by high winds. Shingles that are rated Class H can withstand winds up to 150 miles per hour.

- ◆ Install light-reflective shingles or a white coating on existing shingles to help lower the temperature of your house during the summer and reduce energy consumption.

- ◆ Install photovoltaic shingles to produce solar energy even during a power outage.

- ◆ Use hurricane- and earthquake-resistant nails that are less likely to be pulled out of wood by high winds or tremors.

Mitigate Property Damage & Personal Injury

❑ Apply foam adhesive to the underside of your roof. It helps keep your roof in place during high winds, reducing damage to the roof itself as well as wind and water damage to other parts of the house and its contents due to a failed roof. Foam adhesive also insulates against cold in the winter and heat in the summer and increases protection against fire.

❑ Install hurricane straps or clips to increase the stability of your structure and help prevent the roof from blowing off in high winds.

❑ If you have a barrel-style tile roof, install bird-stops at the roof edges to prevent the buildup of combustible materials.

❑ Install gutter covers to keep combustible materials from collecting in your gutters and downspouts.

Garage

❏ Make sure windows in overhead garage doors and personnel entry doors are double-paned tempered glass, or replace the glass with solid panels for increased security.

❏ Seal gaps around doors to prevent burning embers from entering the space.

❏ Store flammable materials, such as gasoline and chemicals, in proper containers, and store the containers in a fire-resistant cabinet.

❏ Purchase and store fire-retardant gel or foam to apply to the exterior of your home in case of an approaching wildfire.

Other Structures

❏ Locate other structures, such as fences, sheds, and gazebos, at least 50 feet from the house to slow the spread of fire.

Decks

❏ If you are building a new deck, use noncombustible materials. If you use wood, use fire-retardant lumber. Note that the thicker the boards are, the smaller the fire hazard.

❏ Place gravel underneath the deck to discourage plant growth, which can dry out and provide fuel to a fire.

❏ Do not store combustible materials, such as firewood or chemicals, underneath a deck.

❏ Install fine mesh screening along the sides of the deck to prevent combustible debris from being blown in underneath the boards.

❏ Cover gaps around the deck with fine mesh screening to prevent the buildup of combustible debris. If ledger boards are attached to the house without gaps, install flashing as not only a water barrier but also a fire barrier.

Fences & Walls

❑ If you are erecting a new fence or wall, use noncombustible materials. If you use wood, use fire-retardant lumber. (The thicker the boards are, the smaller the fire hazard.) Also consider a design that minimizes the use of combustible materials, such as wood framing with wire mesh in between, rather than all wood, or a chain-link fence interwoven with colored metal or plastic slats for aesthetic value.

❑ Place gravel along the bottom of the fence to discourage plant growth, which can dry out and provide fuel to a fire.

❑ Store combustible materials, such as firewood, away from your house and away from fences or walls.

❑ To prevent landslides on sloped areas, install special retaining fences that create a barrier to hold back rocks and minimize soil erosion and debris flow.

❑ To protect downhill property in cold climates, install special retaining fences that create a barrier to hold back snow to help prevent avalanches.

❑ Install snow fences to keep snow drifts off roads and walkways.

❑ If you live on a lakeshore, build a breakwater or floodwall to prevent flooding.

❑ If you have a stream running across your property, keep the channel dredged and build up the banks to create levees. Plant vegetation to lessen erosion of the embankments to prevent flooding.

LANDSCAPING

❑ Let the grass grow. Roots grow in proportion to the grass blades. The taller the grass is, the longer the roots are, and the better your lawn can tolerate dry conditions during a drought.

❑ Cultivate native, deep-rooted ornamental plants. Indigenous plants have evolved to survive in the climate where they exist. Deep roots help to hold dry soil in place during a drought.

❑ Plant shade trees on your property to lower the temperature around your house during a heat wave.

❑ Use soaker hoses or install a drip-irrigation system to save water by reducing evaporation.

❑ Mulch around plants to hold moisture in the soil.

❑ Stabilize slopes on your property by increasing drainage to reduce the water content of the earth, changing the slope of the hillside, and/or reinforcing the ground with metal anchors, concrete, and other materials. This kind of work is not for amateurs. Consult a geotechnical engineer.

❑ Make sure that an advancing fire doesn't have a direct path to your home through vegetation.

   ❑ Maintain a 50-foot defensible perimeter around your home, using grass, loosely spaced trees and shrubs, and firebreaks such as walkways and driveways.

   ❑ Use nonflammable landscaping materials such as pavers, rocks, and plants with high moisture content.

   ❑ Plant small varieties of vegetation and scatter them in clusters. Vegetation on a flat or slightly sloping lot should be at least 30 feet apart. Vegetation on a steeper slope should be 30 to 60 feet apart.

   ❑ Remove vegetation next to the house and transplant it away from structures.

   ❑ Keep plants near the house pruned and watered. Remove leaves, needles, and other dead plant materials on a regular basis.

   ❑ Plant deciduous trees. Evergreen trees tend to generate more embers than deciduous trees. The wind can easily carry ignited pine cones around your property and spread fire.

   ❑ Consult your local fire officials for recommendations on plant selection and vegetation management to account for slope at your site and winds in your locale.

Before Disaster

Mitigate Property Damage & Personal Injury

Dwelling Interior

Loose Objects

❑ Strap your water heater to wall studs.

❑ If you have a free-standing stove, bolt it to the floor or the wall.

❑ Ensure that light fixtures and ceiling fans are hung securely.

❑ Move pictures, mirrors, and other wall-hangings away from beds.

❑ Bolt shelves and other furniture to wall studs.

❑ Add molding to the edges of open shelves.

❑ Anchor objects to shelves or tables with adhesive or putty.

❑ Install latches on cabinet doors to keep them closed.

❑ Secure electronics such as TV's and computers.

❑ Store hazardous materials in approved containers and place the containers in sturdy fire-resistant cabinets bolted to the wall.

Interior Window Coverings

❑ Install insulated draperies, shades, or blinds on your windows.

❑ Cut plastic sheeting for all exterior openings of your shelter.

Energy Usage

❑ Make sure your house is properly insulated.

❑ Make sure the seals are tight on the refrigerator and freezer.

Filters

❑ Install HEPA filters in your ventilation system and vacuum cleaner.

Mitigate Property Damage & Personal Injury

Electrical

❑ Install smoke detectors in each bedroom and each living space.

❑ Install an interlock or transfer switch on your home's electrical panel to make it safe and easy to convert your power source to your generator.

Plumbing

❑ Insulate your pipes to keep them from freezing.

❑ Use flexible tubing to connect gas appliances to rigid supply lines.

❑ Install backflow valves on all drains.

❑ Install a sump pump with a battery backup.

❑ Keep a gas-powered pump on site, along with fuel to operate it.

❑ Repair leaky faucets.

❑ Attach flow restrictors or aerators to all sink faucets.

❑ Install a low-flow shower head.

❑ Use a high-efficiency water-saving clothes washer and dishwasher.

Safe Room

❑ Create a safe room.

❑ Store your core emergency supplies in the safe room.

Dwelling Exterior

❑ If you have an LP gas tank on your property, secure it against high winds and earthquake tremors.

❑ If your structure is near water, keep sandbags, sand, and shovels ready to go in case the water rises.

❑ Install fire extinguishers outside near sources of fire, such as an outdoor fireplace, fire pit, or grill.

❑ Keep a can of International Orange spray paint on hand.

Security

❑ Make sure your property is well-lit on the outside.

❑ Cut away dense undergrowth that could provide cover for an intruder.

❑ Erect a fence along the perimeter of your property.

❑ Set trip wires that will activate an alarm if anyone breaches the perimeter of your property.

❑ Install solar-powered motion sensors with lights along your property lines and near your dwelling.

❑ Install surveillance cameras along your property lines and near your dwelling.

❑ Install an alarm system with a loud horn on your dwelling. Install sensors on all doors and windows and wire them into the system.

❑ Get watch dogs and attack dogs.

Doors

❑ Install deadbolt locks on all exterior doors.

❑ Install security gates on doorways.

❑ Reinforce exterior doors to keep out projectiles during high winds.

Mitigate Property Damage & Personal Injury

Windows

❏ Install awnings over windows that receive direct sun.

❏ Install dual-pane or triple-pane windows.

❏ To reduce breakability, install laminated glass or apply protective film to standard glass panes.

❏ Install steel bars or alarm mesh screens over windows.

❏ Purchase or fabricate shutters or other temporary covers to fit over doors, windows, vents, and any other openings of your structures.

Roof & Gutters

❏ Use roofing materials that are resistant to hail, wind, fire, and earthquakes, as well as energy-efficient.

❏ Apply foam adhesive to the underside of your roof.

❏ Install hurricane straps or clips to increase the stability of your structure and help prevent the roof from blowing off in high winds.

❏ If you have a barrel-style tile roof, install bird-stops at the roof edges.

❏ Install gutter covers to keep combustible materials from collecting.

Garage

❏ Make sure windows in overhead garage doors and personnel entry doors are double-paned tempered glass, or replace the glass with solid panels for increased security.

❏ Seal gaps around doors to prevent burning embers from entering the space.

❏ Store flammable materials, such as gasoline and chemicals, in proper containers, and store the containers in a fire-resistant cabinet.

❏ Purchase and store fire-retardant gel or foam to apply to the exterior of your home in case of an approaching wildfire.

Other Structures

❑ Locate structures such as fences, sheds, and gazebos at least 50 feet from the house to slow the spread of fire.

❑ If you are building a new deck, use noncombustible materials. If you use wood, use fire-retardant lumber.

❑ Place gravel underneath the deck to discourage plant growth.

❑ Remove combustible materials, such as firewood or chemicals, from underneath decks.

❑ Install fine mesh screening along the sides of the deck to prevent combustible debris from being blown in underneath the boards.

❑ Cover gaps around the deck with fine mesh screening to prevent the buildup of combustible debris.

❑ Use noncombustible materials to build fences or walls. If you use wood, use fire-retardant lumber.

❑ Place gravel along the bottom of the fence to discourage plant growth.

❑ Store combustible materials, such as firewood, away from your house and away from fences or walls.

❑ Install retaining fences on slopes to hold back rocks and minimize soil erosion and debris flow.

❑ To protect downhill property in cold climates, install special retaining fences that create a barrier to hold back snow.

❑ Install snow fences to keep snow drifts off roads and walkways.

❑ If you live on a lakeshore, build a breakwater or floodwall to prevent flooding.

❑ If you have a stream running across your property, dredge the channel and build up the banks to create levees. Plant vegetation to lessen erosion of the embankments.

Landscaping

❑ Cultivate native, deep-rooted ornamental plants.

❑ Plant shade trees on your property.

❑ Use soaker hoses or install a drip-irrigation system.

❑ Mulch around plants.

❑ Stabilize slopes on your property.

❑ Make sure that an advancing fire doesn't have a direct path to your home through vegetation.

   ❑ Maintain a 50-foot defensible perimeter around your home, using grass, loosely spaced trees and shrubs, and firebreaks such as walkways and driveways.

   ❑ Use nonflammable landscaping materials such as pavers, rocks, and plants with high moisture content.

   ❑ Keep plants small and scatter them in clusters. Vegetation on a flat or slightly sloping lot should be at least 30 feet apart. Vegetation on a steeper slope should be 30 to 60 feet apart.

   ❑ Remove any vegetation next to the house and replant it away from the house.

   ❑ Prune and water plants near the house. Remove leaves, needles, and other dead plant materials on a regular basis.

   ❑ Plant deciduous trees. Evergreen trees tend to generate more embers than deciduous trees. The wind can easily carry ignited pine cones around your property and spread fire.

   ❑ Consult your local fire officials for recommendations on plant selection and vegetation management to account for slope at your site and winds in your locale.

Chapter 4

Supplies

This chapter covers the items to keep among your sheltering-in-place supplies and in your evacuation kits. You need sheltering-in-place supplies for your home, your vehicles, and your workplace. You need two kinds of evacuation kits, one to evacuate from home and one to evacuate from work. An evacuation kit is sometimes called a "bug-out bag," a "grab bag," a "go bag," a "blow-out bag," a "GOOD bag" (as in "Get Out Of Dodge"), or a "72-hour kit" (because it holds enough supplies to sustain you for 72 hours). A work evacuation kit is your "get home bag."

The supplies for sheltering-in-place and the evacuation kits are similar, but obviously an evacuation kit must be portable, and it must be packed and ready to go without notice. You may be tempted to use your sheltering-in-place supplies for your evacuation kits. However, if your evacuation supplies aren't packed, you may lose valuable time trying to pack them in an emergency. For this reason, it is wise to have separate supplies for sheltering-in-place and evacuating. In addition, your sheltering-in-place supplies may be standard-sized items, while your evacuation supplies may be travel-sized miniatures. At the very least, keep your core supplies - medical supplies and a minimum amount of water and food for each group member - packed and ready to go. Then if time permits during evacuation, you can pack additional water, food supplies, and other items from your sheltering-in-place storehouse.

The topics in this chapter include:
- water
- food
- sanitation supplies
- medical supplies
- clothing
- bedding & towels
- backpacks
- shelter
- money
- pets

GENERAL GUIDELINES

♦ To free up storage space for emergency supplies, use vacuum-seal bags to store out-of-season clothes, blankets, and sleeping bags. (You know the kind: you use your vacuum cleaner to suck out the air, and your stuff ends up looking flatter than a fritter.).

♦ Seal your emergency supplies in plastic bags to protect them from water, vermin, and contamination from dirt and germs. Double-bag fire-starting materials.

♦ Store your supplies so they're easily accessible.

♦ Store your emergency lighting where it is easily accessible in the dark in case of a power outage. Once you have portable lighting (a flashlight or lantern), you'll be able to see to bring your other supplies out of storage.

♦ Make sure all household members know where the supplies are stored.

♦ Rotate your stock to keep perishable items fresh. This applies to food, water, medications, and batteries.

♦ If you expect to be in a watercraft of any kind (canoe, rowboat, sailboat, etc.) be prepared to capsize. Using a long cord, attach a plastic bottle as a float to your knapsack, duffel bag, or whatever bundle you will be carrying. If you capsize, your bag will stay afloat so you can retrieve it.

♦ For your evacuation kits, pack items that can serve double duty. For instance, a plastic storage container is just a plastic storage container, but a storage container with a shiny metal lid can be used as a reflector to start a fire or signal for help.

♦ The supplies that you need can be found at sporting goods stores, camping stores, outdoor stores, or online.

WATER

The length of time that you can survive without water depends on the outside temperature, your level of activity, and other factors, but even in the best of conditions, survivability without water is only about three days, so having an adequate water supply is vital to your long-term survival.

Prepare for the worst-case scenario: assume that your water supply will be compromised, either because potable water won't flow, or because the water that is available may be contaminated.

Maintaining an adequate water supply can be accomplished through storage of potable water, treatment of contaminated water, or a combination of the two. Since water is one of your most critical needs in a survival situation, this is one area where it is imperative to build redundancy into your plans.

For your sheltering-in-place plan for home, take a three-pronged approach:

- Upgrade and maintain your home's water treatment system so that you will always have potable water as long as water is being pumped.

- Store potable water for short-term needs in case the flow of water is interrupted.

- Have several treatment methods as backups in case the duration of a disaster outlasts your stored supply of potable water.

For sheltering-in-place while away from home or for evacuations, be prepared with portable solutions, such as bottled water, filters, and chemical treatments.

- Store bottles of water in each vehicle.

- Store bottles of water in your desk or locker at work.

- Carry water, portable filters, and purification chemicals with you any time you go hiking, mountain biking, rock climbing, etc. The farther you get from civilization, the more important this becomes.

Treating contaminated water means removing biological contaminants, chemical contaminants, and/or radiological contaminants. Various methods can be used to remove contaminants from water; combining two or more methods results in the most effective treatment against the broadest range of impurities.

Be prepared to treat all contaminated water before using it for drinking, food preparation, teeth brushing, or other hygienic purposes. Consuming water with biological contaminants can quickly lead to waterborne illnesses such as cholera, typhoid, dysentery, and a bunch of other diseases that have names way too long to list here.

Home Water Treatment System

A water treatment system for your home can range from a small cartridge that filters out metals, chemicals, and some bacteria, to a sophisticated reverse osmosis system that filters out virtually all contaminants.

Water treatment devices come in many sizes. A "whole-house" or "point-of-entry" device is installed where the water line enters the house, and it treats all incoming water. A "point-of-use" device is installed where the water is dispensed, and it treats only the water at that dispensing location. It may be an under-the-sink unit, a countertop unit, a screw-on unit installed at the end of a faucet, a refrigerator filter, or a pitcher filter. A point-of-entry device is large and treats several hundred gallons of water per day. A point-of-use device is small and treats only a few gallons per day, typically only enough for drinking purposes.

The initial cost of a point-of-entry device is higher, but it has a substantially longer service life than a point-of-use device. An under-the-sink or countertop unit costs more than a simple faucet filter, but those units also have a longer service life. The overall operational cost of a point-of-entry device is higher than a point-of-use device, but a point-of-entry device treats a much higher volume of water. The per-gallon cost of a point-of-entry device is generally lower than a point-of-use device.

One advantage of filtering your own water is that it reduces the need for bottled water and therefore reduces plastic waste.

Look for a filtering system that removes all of the following:

◆ microbial cysts that are resistant to other methods of disinfection

◆ heavy metals such as lead and mercury

◆ industrial pollutants from factories

◆ pharmaceuticals (legal and illegal!) that are flushed down the drain

◆ by-products of chlorine disinfection (total trihalomethanes, or TTHMs)

If your home has a reverse osmosis system, you most likely will have a reliable supply of safe water as long as the water continues to flow. If the water ceases to flow for any reason, you will have to rely on stored water for your needs.

Regardless of the water treatment system you use, it must be properly maintained to be effective. An improperly maintained system may worsen the water quality by adding contaminants back into the water rather than removing them.

Quantity of Stored Water Needed

For sheltering-in-place at home, keep a two-week supply for each person, allowing one gallon per person per day (½ gallon for drinking + ½ gallon for cooking and sanitation).

1 gallon/person x _____ people x 14 days = _____ gallons total

Children, pregnant women, nursing mothers, the sick, and the elderly may require more. Hot environments and increased physical activity may also increase the amount of water needed. Consuming juice, prepared drinks, soup, and high moisture foods will slightly reduce the amount of water you will need.

Allow one quart per day for each dog or cat.

1 quart/pet x _____ pets x 14 days = _____ quarts total

_____ quarts / 4 = _____ gallons total

For sheltering-in-place in your vehicle or at work, keep a three-day supply, allowing ½ gallon per day for drinking.

For evacuation, pack a three-day supply of bottled water for each person, allowing ½ gallon per person per day for drinking. To meet your water needs beyond that, pack portable treatments such as carbon filters, iodine, or chlorine, discussed later in this chapter.

Water Sources

Tap Water From A Public Source

Communities that supply water to the public are required to regularly test for bacteria and deliver water that meets EPA (Environmental Protection Agency) drinking-water standards. If your house taps into a public water supply, this water is presumed safe for storage before a disaster occurs. However, because it does contain some bacteria, treating it is recommended to further reduce the level of bacteria before long-term storage.

To treat water for storage, use liquid household chlorine bleach that contains 5.25 % sodium hypochlorite. Do not use bleach with additives, such as added cleaners or scents.

1. Using a sterile medicine dropper, add 16 drops of bleach per gallon of water and stir.

2. Allow the treated water to stand for 30 minutes.

3. If the odor of chlorine is not detectable after 30 minutes, repeat the process until a slight odor of chlorine is present.

4. Pour into clean containers, cap the containers, and label them with the contents and date.

Tap Water From A Private Source

Drinking water drawn from private water supplies - individual wells and springs - should be tested for bacteria at least annually, as well as any time you notice a change in the taste, odor, or appearance of the water. The risk of contamination depends on the quality of your well construction, your diligence in maintaining it, the quality of the aquifer from which water is drawn, and nearby activities such as agricultural or industrial uses.

To help safeguard your water supply:

♦ Keep pet waste, pesticides, gasoline, oil, and other chemicals off the ground and at least 100 feet away from your well.

♦ Perform regular well disinfections:

1. Pour chlorine bleach down the sides of the well and into the water.

2. Connect a hose to a faucet and run water back into the well for 30 minutes.

3. Open all faucets in the house and run water until you can smell chlorine.

4. Close all faucets and allow the chlorinated water to stand in the pipes for 10 to 12 hours.

5. Seal all openings into the well.

6. Open all faucets and run water until the chlorine is flushed from the system.

7. Use a point-of-entry or point-of-use carbon filter to remove the by-products of chlorine disinfection (total trihalomethanes, or TTHMs).

♦ Maintain your septic system.

♦ Use water efficiently to allow the tank and drain field to work properly. Fix leaky faucets. Use high-efficiency toilets, showerheads, faucets, washing machines, and dishwashers. Run the clothes washer and dishwasher only when full. Limit the use of the garbage disposal.

♦ Have the septic system professionally inspected and have the tank pumped out regularly, generally every one to three years, depending on the size and kind of system you have and the number of people using the system.

♦ Don't dispose of hazardous wastes through sinks or toilets. The only water going down the sink or shower drains should be wastewater from washing your body, brushing your teeth, washing food, washing dishes, or washing clothes. The only things going down the toilet should be human waste and toilet paper. Avoid putting paper towels, feminine hygiene products, diapers, cotton swabs, dental floss, condoms, cigarette butts, coffee grounds, cat litter, household chemicals, pesticides, gasoline, oil, antifreeze, or paint in any drain or toilet.

♦ Protect your drain field.

  * Plant nothing but grass over your septic system. Roots from trees and shrubs can clog and damage the drain field.

  * Shield the drain field from being flooded with excessive water, as this slows or stops treatment processes and can cause plumbing fixtures to clog. Stagger the use of the dishwasher and clothes washer to spread water usage throughout the week. Keep roof drains, sump drains, and other drainage systems away from the septic drain field.

  * Don't drive or park vehicles over any part of your septic system. Doing so can damage the piping or tank or compact the soil in your drain field.

If you have a whole-house treatment system that includes a process such as reverse osmosis or distillation, your water most likely will be safe to store if the system was installed correctly and has been properly maintained.

Even if you don't have a reverse osmosis or distillation system, if your well water is safe for day-to-day usage, it is presumed safe for storage before a disaster occurs. However, like municipal water, it does contain some bacteria, so treating it is recommended to further reduce the level of bacteria before long-term storage. (See Tap Water From A Public Source above.) If you doubt the quality of your well water, purchase bottled water for long-term storage.

Commercially Bottled Water

Water sold in bottles ranges from a few ounces to the five-gallon size used with bottled-water dispensers. Such water may be labeled "spring water," "distilled water," "purified water," "de-ionized water," or other descriptions.

Look for a seal from the IBWA (International Bottled Water Association) or NSF (National Sanitation Foundation). These organizations require periodic inspection and testing of bottling facilities. Purchase unopened bottles only.

Vended Water

Water vending machines allow consumers to fill their own containers with treated city water. The vendor typically provides additional treatment beyond what is done by the city. Vended water is regulated by the Food and Drug Administration, which requires that such water come from an approved public water supply, which in turn is regulated by the Environmental Protection Agency. This assures that the water itself is safe, but the vending machine (and your own container!) must also be sanitary in order for the vended water to be clean enough to drink.

Collected Rain Water

Collect rainwater in barrels or a cistern (unless prohibited by local ordinances). Treat it before drinking to get rid of any impurities.

Waterbeds

Materials used in waterbeds are not approved for food storage, and some waterbed materials contain toxic chemicals. If you are going to use a waterbed as an emergency water reservoir, drain it yearly and refill it with fresh water containing ¼ cup of bleach per 120 gallons of water. Do not add any other chemicals, including algaecides. Plan to boil the water before using it, or use it only for flushing toilets.

Water Containers

While the water itself must be safe to drink, the containers used to collect and store the water must also be clean. Any contamination in a container will render the water unsafe to drink. The best way to store potable water depends on the configuration of your storage space and how strong the members of your group are.

Individual-serving-size bottles are easy to handle, but they take up a lot of room and produce a lot of plastic waste to dispose of.

> 8-ounce bottle x 16 bottles = 1 gallon (one-day supply for one person)
> 16 bottles x 14 days = 224 bottles (two-week supply for one person)

Five-gallon bottles take up less room overall, but they're heavy to lift. A 55-gallon drum takes up the least amount of room by volume, but is too heavy to move; you must be able to rig it with a pump to empty and refill the drum every six months to keep the water fresh. And although a 55-gallon drum provides the most efficient storage, it takes up a large amount of space in one place, compared to small bottles that can be stashed in nooks and crannies throughout the house.

Another way to store a large volume of water is to collect rain water in a cistern. For information on how to build a cistern, search online, visit the library, or consult a professional contractor. (Check local ordinances first.)

If you bottle your own water, store it in food-grade plastic with tight fitting lids. You can buy new plastic containers or reuse clean soda and juice bottles and food jars, but do not reuse plastic milk jugs, as it is difficult to remove the protein and fat residues that allow bacteria to grow. If you bottle your own water and treat it with chlorine, do not store it in metal containers, as chlorine is corrosive to most metals.

Do not reuse any container that has held a toxic substance, as trace amounts may remain. Other containers not labeled for food storage could also release harmful chemicals into the water. Although chlorine bleach can be used to sterilize water, bleach bottles or other plastic bottles are not recommended for water storage because chlorine can react with plastic long-term to produce harmful chemical compounds. Containers that are not approved for food storage can be used to store water for flushing toilets or other uses that don't require potable water. Avoid using containers that will disintegrate or break, such as paper cartons or glass bottles.

Water Storage

Store containers in a cool, dry, dark place.

Plastic degrades over time, so store plastic containers away from heat and light to prevent leakage.

Hydrocarbon vapors can penetrate polyethylene plastics, so store plastic containers away from gasoline, kerosene, pesticides, or other carbon-based substances.

A gallon of water weighs over eight pounds. Make sure shelves and floors are strong enough to support the weight.

If you have room, store some water in the freezer. If you lose power, the frozen water will help keep foods frozen for a longer period of time. Water expands as it freezes, so as you fill your container with water, leave a couple of inches of air space at the top to keep the container from cracking.

Shelf Life of Water & Usage of Stored Water

Replace home-bottled water every six months. Replace unopened commercially bottled water every twelve months. Rotate it out of storage and use it at regular intervals.

If you use your stored water during an emergency, practice standard sanitation to keep your water safe and reduce the exposure to contamination. Open and use one container at a time. Wash your hands before handling containers. Keep used utensils away from the container opening. Don't drink directly out of the containers.

If water is cloudy or has a smell other than the odor of chlorine, it must be re-treated before using it.

Water that has been disinfected with chlorine should be run through a carbon filter to remove the by-products of chlorine disinfection (total trihalomethanes, or TTHMs) before using it.

Water stored for a long time may taste flat. To improve the taste, restore oxygen to it by pouring it back and forth from one clean container to another several times.

Short-term Water Treatment

Stored water occupies a lot of space. Be prepared to treat contaminated tap water or surface water to make it potable as an alternative to stockpiling a large volume of potable water and as a backup in case you exhaust your supply of potable water during a crisis.

Treatment of contaminated water involves the removal of solid debris (sticks, leaves, gravel, sand, and soil), biological contaminants, chemical contaminants, and/or radioactive materials. Desalination of seawater may also be necessary.

Water can be treated by filtration, heat sterilization, ultraviolet radiation, solar disinfection, chemical disinfection, distillation, reverse osmosis, and forward osmosis. The method you choose depends on the kind of contaminants you are trying to eliminate and the resources you have available. A combination of two or more methods may be required to obtain potable water.

The following methods on the next few pages can be used short-term while sheltering-in-place at home or away from home or during a temporary evacuation.

If you experience an apocalyptic situation – for example, your municipal water supply ceases to function on a permanent basis, or you are forced to permanently relocate and rebuild on your own – you will need a continuous purification system with gravel, sand filters, a pump, piping, holding tanks, and other components. For more information, see the chapter entitled "Apocalypse Plan."

Filtration

Filtration of water on a short-term basis includes the use of paper, cloth, ceramic, or polymer filters that create physical barriers, and carbon filters that work through adsorption. Low-tech paper or cloth filters can be whatever you have available: coffee filter, tea bag, paper towel, printer paper, construction paper, cheesecloth, dish towel, tee shirt, sheet, etc. High-tech ceramic and polymer filters and carbon filters are sold in disposable cartridges.

Filters sold in cartridges weigh from a few ounces to more than a pound, so some are easier to carry than others. Filter lifetime is affected by the size and quantity of particles in the water. Filters clog from the particles being screened as well as the growth of organisms in the filter medium. In addition, droplets of retained water may freeze and cause the filter element to crack in cold weather.

Small-pore mechanical filters of 0.1 microns can effectively screen out bacteria, but viruses are small enough to pass through, so additional treatment must be used in conjunction with filtration in order to neutralize all biological contamination

The pro's and con's of mechanical filters (used alone):
♦ effective at removing solid debris
♦ effective against some biological contaminants, depending on size
♦ ineffective against chemical contamination
♦ effective against some nuclear contamination, depending on size
♦ may be bulkier than chemical disinfectants
♦ may be costlier than chemical disinfectants

An activated carbon filter is typically used to complement other purification methods and is commonly used after mechanical filtering and chlorination. It removes chemical compounds that cannot be removed by reverse osmosis or distillation and chemical compounds referred to as disinfection by-products that occur when chlorine reacts with organic matter in water. . Ceramic and polymer filters are frequently packaged with a carbon filter.

The pro's and con's of carbon filters:
♦ ineffective against biological contaminants
♦ effective against chemical contamination
♦ ineffective against nuclear contamination
♦ improve taste of filtered water

Heat Sterilization

Heating water until it boils is all that is necessary to kill germs. Water temperatures above 185°F kill all pathogens within a few minutes. By the time water reaches the boiling point of 212°F, it has been hot enough long enough to destroy any organisms that can make you sick. In addition, after the water is removed from the heat source, it takes several more minutes for the water to cool enough to drink, during which time it continues to remain hot enough to destroy pathogens. As long as you heat water until it reaches a rolling boil, you've heated it long enough. Boiling it any longer is a waste of fuel.

Boiled water may taste "flat." To improve the taste, add oxygen to the water by pouring it back and forth between two clean containers. This technique also improves the taste of stored water.

The pro's and con's of heat sterilization:
♦ ineffective at removing solid debris
♦ effective against biological contaminants
♦ ineffective against chemical contamination
♦ ineffective against nuclear contamination
♦ requires fuel and an appropriate heating container
♦ relatively inexpensive, depending on cost of fuel
♦ time-consuming due to heating and cooling period
♦ makes water taste "flat"

Ultraviolet (UV) Radiation

Ultraviolet radiation inactivates bacteria without the use of heat or chemical additives. A low-pressure mercury vapor lamp, also called a germicidal lamp, provides a cost-effective and efficient source of short-wave ultraviolet energy.

The effectiveness of UV radiation depends on both the length of time and the intensity of the radiation to which an organism is exposed. A short exposure time at high intensity is as effective as a long exposure time at low intensity.

The radiation must strike a microorganism to inactivate it. The water must be clear enough to allow transmission of an adequate amount of UV energy. If the water is muddy, filtering is required to remove dirt and other debris before disinfection can take place.

The pro's and con's of UV radiation:
♦   ineffective at removing solid debris
♦   effective against biological contaminants
♦   ineffective against chemical contamination
♦   ineffective against nuclear contamination
♦   requires a power source to operate the lamp
♦   may be bulkier than chemical disinfectants
♦   initial cost is higher than chemical disinfectants

Solar Disinfection

Solar disinfection is a method of sterilizing water using transparent PET (polyester) bottles and sunlight, destroying organisms by heat and radiation from the sun. A water-filled PET bottle is left in full sunlight for six hours, or if only partial sunlight is available, for two days. Bottles heat faster and to higher temperatures if they are placed on a sloped corrugated metal roof facing the sun. This method kills almost all microbes that may be present.

Solar disinfection is an effective method for treating water when fuel or heating vessels are unavailable. It is economical and environmentally friendly in the sense that you don't consume fuel or use harsh chemicals, but it does create plastic waste to dispose of.

Solar disinfection is time-consuming and the amount of potable water produced is limited by the number of bottles that are available.
If the water is muddy, filtering is required to remove dirt and other debris before solar disinfection can take place.

The pro's and con's of solar disinfection:
♦ ineffective at removing solid debris
♦ effective against most, but not all, biological contaminants
♦ ineffective against chemical contamination
♦ ineffective against nuclear contamination
♦ requires transparent polyethylene bottles
♦ relatively inexpensive
♦ time-consuming due to waiting period

Chemical Disinfection - Iodine

Iodine is available as a liquid and as a solid, in the form of tablets or crystals. In an emergency, you can use the iodine from your first-aid kit.

Iodine kills most microorganisms, but not all. Allow water treated with iodine to sit for at least 30 minutes to achieve the highest kill rate. The colder the water, the longer you have to wait.

To use the crystal form, a couple of ounces of water is added to a bottle of crystals. Once the water is saturated with iodine, the iodine-saturated water (but not the iodine crystals) is added to the container of water to be purified. The iodine crystals can be reused.

Liquid iodine has a relatively long shelf life. Iodine tablets are effective indefinitely until the storage container is opened; after the container is opened, the stated shelf life is three months. Iodine crystals have a long shelf life as long as they are not left exposed to air.

Iodine-treated water is not suitable for people who are allergic to iodine, have thyroid disease, or are pregnant.

Iodine tablets and crystals are small and lightweight, making them portable and easy to store.

For treating a large volume of water, iodine crystals are cheaper than iodine tablets.

To avoid the objectionable taste of iodine, Vitamin C can be added to the water after it has been disinfected.

The pro's and con's of iodine:
♦ ineffective at removing solid debris
♦ effective against most, but not all, biological contaminants
♦ ineffective against chemical contamination
♦ ineffective against nuclear contamination
♦ portable
♦ relatively inexpensive
♦ time-consuming due to waiting period
♦ long shelf life if handled properly
♦ leaves unpleasant taste in water unless treated with vitamin C

Chemical Disinfection – Chlorine

Chlorine is available in liquid and tablet form.

Ordinary household chlorine bleach, which typically contains a solution of 5% sodium hypochlorite, can be used to disinfect water. Water is treated by stirring in 16 drops of bleach per gallon of water and letting it stand for 30 minutes. Use only plain liquid bleach. Do not use scented bleaches, color-safe bleaches, or bleaches with added cleaners.

Chlorine is more effective than iodine as a disinfectant, but it doesn't kill all microorganisms.

Chlorine tablets have a shelf life of about six months, so they have to be replaced periodically. Liquid chlorine bleach is readily available and relatively inexpensive, but liquid chlorine bleach also degrades with age.

TTHMs are total trihalomethanes, chemical compounds referred to as disinfection by-products. They occur when chlorine reacts with organic matter in water, and may have adverse health effects. The easiest way to reduce or eliminate TTHMs in drinking water that has been treated with chlorine is to use a carbon filter afterwards. When using a filter, verify that it is certified to remove TTHMs and follow replacement instructions recommended by the manufacturer. Note that the health risks from biological contaminants outweigh the risks from TTHMs. So if you must use chlorine to disinfect your water, but you don't have a carbon filter to remove the TTHMs afterwards, go ahead and use the chlorine anyway; even if you don't have a carbon filter to remove the TTHMs, it's better to use chlorine alone to remove bacteria than not use anything at all.

The pro's and con's of chlorine:
♦   ineffective at removing solid debris
♦   effective against most, but not all, biological contaminants
♦   ineffective against chemical contamination
♦   ineffective against nuclear contamination
♦   tablets are very portable; liquid is bulky
♦   relatively inexpensive
♦   readily available
♦   time-consuming due to waiting period
♦   produces disinfection by-products that should be removed
♦   leaves objectionable taste in water unless chlorine is removed

Distillation

Distillation is accomplished by vaporizing water and then condensing the vapor back into a liquid that is relatively free of impurities.

One way to do this is to use a pot with a lid. Pour the contaminated water into the pot about halfway. Tie a cup to the underneath side of the lid, with the cup upright and the lid on top. Place the lid over the pot, with the cup underneath hanging right-side-up over the water (not in the water). Heat the water to boiling. The water that drips from the lid into the cup is distilled. This method requires a heat source, and is a painfully slow process to produce a small amount of potable water.

If you don't have a lid, a variation on this method is to build a frame and position a piece of plastic over the pot in an inverted "V" so that steam from the pot condenses on the underneath side of the plastic and water runs down and drips into a container at the end of the plastic.

If you don't have a fuel source, a solar still is an alternate way to distill water. Place a small bowl inside a larger bowl with high sides (the sides of the large bowl must be higher than the small bowl). Pour the contaminated water into the large bowl, without letting any spill into the small bowl. Cover the large bowl with plastic wrap. Place a coin or other small object on top of the plastic wrap, directly over the small bowl, to give the plastic wrap a funnel or V shape. Do not let the plastic wrap touch the small bowl. Leave the bowls in bright sunlight for a few hours. Condensation will form on the plastic wrap. The water that drips from the plastic wrap into the small bowl is distilled. You can speed up the process by using a dark-colored bowl to absorb more heat from the sun, or by placing aluminum foil around the bowl to direct sunlight onto the water.

In a pit-type solar still, a V-shaped pit is dug into the soil, and a piece of plastic is used to cover the hole, with a weight (such as a rock) in the middle to give the plastic angled sides. (An alternate design is to mound dirt into piles to create a "hole.") The heat of the sun draws moisture out of the soil, and water condenses on the underneath side of the plastic and drips down from the weighted low point into a container.

All of these methods require plastic sheeting or some other "lid," a container to catch the distilled water, and optionally, a drinking tube; commercially packaged kits are also available. All of these variations are painfully slow at producing a small amount of potable water.

Distillation may be the only way to obtain water in a dry environment such as a desert.

Distillation is very effective at removing many kinds of contaminants, but it removes beneficial minerals as well as harmful ones.

The pro's and con's of distillation:
♦ effective at removing solid debris
♦ effective against biological contaminants
♦ effective against some chemical contaminants
♦ effective against nuclear contamination
♦ produces only a small amount of potable water
♦ expensive because of fuel use, unless using solar energy
♦ time-consuming to process
♦ removes beneficial minerals as well as harmful ones

Reverse Osmosis

In this process, water under pressure is forced through a semi-permeable membrane that allows water molecules to pass but inhibits the passage of contaminants with a larger molecular structure. Basic components of the system include a mechanical filter to remove solid debris, the reverse-osmosis unit containing the membrane, an activated carbon filter to remove residual chemicals, a storage tank, a wastewater drain, and valves to control the flow of water. .

These systems are very effective at removing many kinds of contaminants, but they also remove beneficial minerals as well as harmful ones. They have a high upfront cost compared to other water treatment methods, but over the long term, they can be the most cost-effective way to produce an adequate quantity of potable water. The life spans of the filters and membrane depend on the degree of contamination of the water and the quantity of water being treated.

Since reverse-osmosis membranes are very restrictive, these systems tend to have slow flow rates and may produce a smaller quantity of clean water than what you are accustomed to consuming.

Another disadvantage of reverse osmosis is the potentially large quantity of contaminated wastewater that is generated. The quantity generated depends mostly on the pressure difference across the membrane. The larger the pressure difference, the less waste you will have.

The pro's and con's of reverse osmosis:
♦   effective at removing solid debris
♦   effective against biological contaminants
♦   effective against chemical contamination (if carbon filter is used)
♦   effective against nuclear contamination
♦   expensive to install system
♦   removes beneficial minerals as well as harmful ones

Desalination/Forward Osmosis

A whole-house desalination system would be prohibitively expensive and impractical, and unnecessary in most parts of the country. However, if you live near saltwater, having a backup system to produce fresh water from seawater should be a part of your emergency preparedness plan. Whether you tap into a municipal water supply or a private well, your source could become contaminated, and desalination of seawater could be your only option for survival.

Portable self-contained packs can produce potable water from either seawater or brackish marsh water as well as contaminated surface water and even urine. These pouches come as single-use or multiple-use systems.

Other forward-osmosis products include backpack-style or larger vehicle-mounted reservoirs that work like the pouches, but produce a larger quantity of potable water.

Originally developed for military use and space exploration, these systems are available online and at outdoor-supply stores.

The pro's and con's of portable forward-osmosis systems:
♦   effective at removing solid debris (depending on design)
♦   effective against biological contaminants
♦   effective against some chemical contaminants
♦   effective against nuclear contamination
♦   expensive relative to volume of potable water produced
♦   removes beneficial minerals as well as harmful ones

FOOD

Quantity

For sheltering-in-place at home, keep at least a two-week supply of food for each group member. If you want to prepare for an apocalyptic event, you will need to store enough food to last several months or even years.

For sheltering-in-place in your vehicle or at work, keep a three-day supply of nonperishable food.

For evacuation, pack a three-day supply of nonperishable food for each group member.

Sources

Do not plan to rely on grocery stores for your provisions during an emergency. You may not be able to reach the grocery, and even if you can, most grocery shelves would be wiped out in only a few days if they are not able to restock.

Store what you eat. As a general rule, stock the foods that you normally consume. Don't stock foods that you don't want to eat. If a disaster strikes, you're going to have plenty of stuff to complain about.   Don't make yourself even more miserable by forcing yourself and your family to eat foods you don't like. However, for long-term storage, include dried foods, even if these items are not what you would usually consume.

In general, select foods with a long shelf life that require no refrigeration, little or no preparation, and little or no water. Canned products are good choices and provide a variety of foods: milk, meats, fruits, vegetables, and beans.

Select high-energy foods, such as energy bars used by sports participants. These can be found at sporting-goods stores or the nutritional-supplements section of grocery stores.

Store staples such as flour and corn meal only if you can reasonably expect to use them. If you don't know how to cook from scratch, now is a good time to learn!

Another alternative is the MRE (Meal, Ready-to-Eat), a compact, self-contained, individual ration. These self-heating meals are shelf-stable kits of cooked food along with water and a specially treated heating pad. When you're ready to eat the meal, you pour the water on the pad to produce a chemical reaction that creates heat to warm the food. This technology was originally developed by the government with your tax dollars, so think of it as a return on your investment. Millions of MREs have been consumed by soldiers, refugees, and sportsmen. To say these are not gourmet meals is an understatement. On the upside, they require no refrigeration, they can provide a hot meal in an environment lacking amenities, and they have a long shelf life. Various brands of self-heating meals are available in grocery stores, sporting goods stores, and online.

Dried food has several advantages: it has a long shelf life, it requires no refrigeration, and its reduced weight and bulk make it easy to store for sheltering-in-place and easy to carry during an evacuation. However, many dried foods will need to be reconstituted with water in order to be palatable. Drying preserves food by removing the water content, thus inhibiting the growth of microorganisms and slowing decay. Water can be removed by evaporation, as in air drying, or by freeze-drying, wherein food is first frozen and then water is removed by sublimation. Dried food is easily reconstituted with water as long as you have water available.

Groceries carry dried products such as powdered milk and other drinks, beef jerky, dehydrated potatoes, and fruits such as raisins, prunes, banana chips, and so forth. Other dried products can be found at camping or sporting-goods stores. Or use a food dehydrator to make your own dried food.

Shelf Life

Eat what you store. Eat the provisions in your stockpile on a regular basis. By rotating your stock and continually replenishing your warehouse, you'll avoid waste and keep your stored foods fresh.

To build up your supplies, use a weekly, monthly, or quarterly shopping schedule. Once you have enough food in storage, start rotating the oldest goods into your pantry for current use. For instance, when you buy a can of soup, put the new can in the back of your stored goods and move all of the other cans forward one space, putting the oldest can in front so it will be used next. Continually use the items with the earliest expiration dates and replace them with new to keep your stored food supply as fresh as possible.

The following factors affect the shelf-life of packaged food (bagged, canned, and bottled):

▶ **Light**
Store food in the dark.

▶ **Temperature**
Keep food cool. Store it at room temperature, 70° F or below.

▶ **Moisture**
Store food where it will stay dry. Keep it up off the floor.

▶ **Vermin**
Wrap food in plastic bags and put it in plastic totes.
Keep it up off the floor.

Accessories

If you store canned food, be sure to have a manual can opener.

To heat food, be prepared to use canned cooking fuel or another heat source.

For more information on cooking utensils and energy sources, see the "Cooking" topic in the chapter entitled "Tools and Equipment."

SANITATION SUPPLIES

Sanitation supplies include products for personal hygiene (toothpaste, soap, etc.) as well as products to clean cooking and eating utensils, clothing, and bedding. You must also store supplies to clean your environment (toilets!) and remove vermin-attracting garbage and trash.

If you don't observe proper sanitation practices, you'll need more medical supplies, i.e., those used to fight infection. You choose.

MEDICAL SUPPLIES & EQUIPMENT

Medical supplies and equipment can include:

- prescription drugs that you take on a regular basis
- over-the-counter medicines that you take on a regular basis
- nutritional supplements
- disposable supplies, such as blood monitoring/testing supplies, syringes and needles, ostomy supplies, urological supplies, etc.
- prosthetic/orthotic devices
- dental appliances
- eyeglasses, contact lenses, and lens care supplies
- hearing aids
- wheelchairs, lifts, canes, and other durable medical equipment
- first aid kit
- emergency warming blankets
- cooling vest

On your next doctor's visit, ask for two extra prescriptions for each drug that you take. Have one extra prescription filled and put a 30-day supply of the drug in your stockpile. Keep the second extra script with your important papers, to carry with you in case you need to evacuate. As you have prescriptions renewed, rotate your inventory, i.e., use the oldest first and put the newest at the back of the line.

Both over-the-counter and prescription medicines have expiration dates on the packaging, but the medication may be effective even after the stated date. Ask your pharmacist about the shelf life of medications that you take. It won't do you any good to stockpile two years' worth of medicine if it becomes ineffective by the time you might need to use it. Stock only as much as can be used before the end of its effectiveness.

If you have a power wheelchair, keep a spare battery charged up. Also have a manual wheelchair as a spare in case electricity is unavailable for recharging your batteries.

CLOTHING

To prepare for evacuation in case of an emergency, pack a variety of clothing so you can be comfortable in any climate and terrain. If you are taking a trip, wear or pack clothing that is suited to the climate, terrain, and activities that you expect to experience.

Rotate your clothes so that if you get wet, you will always have something dry to put on. Pack your spares in plastic bags to keep them dry.

Think of the specific kinds of gear you may need for each part of your body:

- head
- eyes
- ears
- nose & mouth
- torso, arms, & legs
- hands & fingers
- feet

You need to stay warm in cold weather and cool in hot weather.

You need to protect all areas of your body from injury.

Headgear

For wet environments, pack headgear that is waterproof.

For cold environments, pack a head covering that can be pulled down over your entire face, such as a ski mask. Include a scarf to wrap around your neck.

For desert environments, pack a wide-brimmed, vented hat or a square piece of lightweight cloth that can be draped over your head and shoulders and wrapped around your face to protect you from the sun and sand.

Eye Wear

Protect your eyes from the sun with sunglasses and a broad-brimmed hat.

Protect your eyes from sand and water with goggles.

Include a sweatband to keep perspiration out of your eyes.

Ear Wear

For cold climates, protect your ears with stocking hats, caps with flaps, or thermal earmuffs.

Masks

Disposable dust masks such as those sold at hardware stores effectively filter only large particles and are therefore not recommended for protection in a biological, chemical, or nuclear emergency. They do offer some protection in dust storms.

Any mask that you use for respiratory protection should state that it is approved by NIOSH (National Institute for Occupational Safety and Health).

N95 disposable respiratory masks filter about 95% of particles 0.3 microns and larger and provide good protection against biological threats.

N100 disposable respiratory masks filter almost 100% of particles 0.3 microns and larger and provide better protection against biological and radiological threats.

Only gas masks can effectively filter chemical agents. Since they restrict breathing, they can harm an untrained user, and are therefore not recommended for the average consumer.

If you expect to be in a water environment, include a snorkeling mask in your gear.

Jackets, Vests, Shirts, & Pants

In hot climates, wear light-colored, lightweight, loose-fitting clothing.

In cooler climates at high elevations and/or high latitudes, wear clothes in layers and protect all extremities from the cold. Thermal underwear, flannel-lined or fleece-lined jeans or workpants, leggings, and leg warmers provide additional layers of warmth. Battery-heated jackets, vests, and pants offer extra protection in extreme cold.

A basic jacket in breathable fabric will keep you dry and warm and reduce the amount of sweat you produce, in turn reducing the amount of water you need to consume. It should have large pockets, storm flaps, and a hood. A rainproof shell with a zip-out lining offers versatility for a range of climate conditions.

Cooling vests can be worn to keep you cool while doing strenuous work in hot conditions. They can also be used to cool the core body temperature of someone who is suffering from heat exhaustion.

A tactical vest has pockets and rings that allow you to carry ammunition, a flashlight, flares, canisters of water purification tablets or medications, and other small survival gear.

Pack pants that are comfortable for walking. Lightweight material such as cotton dries quickly. Pants with zip-off legs can be worn throughout the day as the temperature rises and falls. Cargo pants provide extra pockets for carrying gear. Brush pants and chaps offer extra protection in heavy underbrush. Compression shirts and pants aid circulation.

Rain wear can be anything from a thin poncho that folds up and fits in your pocket, to a slicker, to heavy-duty foul weather gear. Waterproof pants need to fit easily over your other gear.

Jackets, shirts, and pants come in a variety of colors, fabrics, and styles to meet any need. Specialty clothes can be found at outdoor stores. Marine stores specialize in waterproof gear.

Gloves

Gloves are made for every purpose you can think of. They can protect you from cold, heat, water, chemicals, and sharp objects, and can prevent frostbite, burns, blisters, broken nails, cuts, and shocks.

Gloves can be made of leather, wool, cotton, rubber, or synthetic fibers. They can be unlined or lined. Linings can provide insulation and wick away perspiration to keep your hands warm and dry. Battery-heated gloves provide even more warmth. Mittens keep your hands warmer than gloves.

Mesh fabric provides ventilation. Long cuffs and reinforced palms, fingers, and knuckles provide extra protection. Open fingertips can give you the nimbleness you need to perform fine tasks while still protecting the rest of your hands. Gloves are also available with mesh fingertips for operating touch screens.

Disposable gloves protect patient and caregiver from cross-contamination when applying first aid or providing nursing care to the sick. They are also useful for handling substances such as permanent glue.

Heat-resistant gloves provide protection for cooking over an open fire, welding, forging, or other work with very hot materials. Cryogenic gloves provide protection in an extremely cold environment.

Puncture-resistant and cut-resistant gloves are coated to protect against sharp and pointed objects such blades, needles, and glass. Rubber gloves provide protection when working with electricity.

The glove you select for any activity should provide maximum protection while maintaining the level of dexterity you need for the task.

Socks

Socks come in all lengths - ankle, mid-calf, knee, and thigh – and are designed for many different purposes. Being in a survival situation may mean you'll be walking a lot, so one of the most useful kinds of socks are hiking socks, designed to provide warmth, dryness, cushioning, and abrasion resistance.

Hiking socks come in a variety of weights to suit different conditions.

Liners are designed to be worn next to your skin under other socks. They are made of thin, lightweight fabric that wicks perspiration away from your skin to keep your feet dry, and they limit abrasion from outer socks.

Lightweight hiking socks are relatively thin and are well suited for warm conditions and easy walking. They usually provide adequate wicking performance and comfort and can be worn with or without liners.

Mid-weight hiking socks are thick and warm and well suited for moderate to cold conditions. They provide reliable cushioning, and sometimes have extra padding in the high-impact areas of the heel and the ball of the foot. They should be worn with liners.

Heavyweight hiking socks are the thickest, warmest and most cushioned. They are well suited for extremely cold temperatures and rough terrain. They should be worn with liners.

Hiking socks can be made of silk, wool, cotton, or synthetic fibers.

Silk is comfortable and lightweight and provides reliable wicking and good insulation, but it is not as durable as other fibers.

Wool is cushioning, warm, and retains heat when wet, but it can irritate your skin and can take a long time to dry, and may quickly become threadbare if not blended with other fibers.

Cotton is comfortable when dry, but has poor wicking properties; since it absorbs moisture, it provides no insulation when wet, and because it is thin, it provides little protection against blisters.

Synthetic fibers are typically blended with natural fibers to improve durability and the wicking and insulating properties of the fabric, as well as to make it less abrasive and quicker to dry. Many hiking socks include elastic materials to help the fabric maintain its shape and minimize bunching.

Other special-purpose socks may come in handy in your survival kits.

Running socks are designed to allow ventilation and wicking of moisture to keep your feet cool and dry.

Electric socks use low-voltage batteries to heat socks and keep your feet warm, but they work only as long as the batteries can hold a charge. In addition, you must make sure the design allows the batteries to fit underneath your pants and inside your boots.

Compression socks are designed to improve circulation and reduce the risk of blood clots. They are frequently recommended for people with diabetes, varicose veins, and deep vein thrombosis, as well as patients recovering from surgery and pregnant women.

Nonskid socks can help prevent slips and falls for people who are unable to wear shoes.

Flame-resistant socks provide protection while fighting a fire or in any environment with a risk of burn injuries from flame, extreme heat, or ignition or where molten metal can penetrate protective outer garments or footwear.

Wear and pack socks that are suited to the climate, terrain, and activities that you expect to be involved in, and that allow your shoes or boots to fit properly.

Footwear

Choose footwear that is likely to be useful to you in an emergency, taking into consideration the terrain and climate you can expect to be in. In an emergency, you may have to walk a lot over mixed terrain in changing weather conditions, so hiking boots should be an essential item in your survival kit. Select comfortable boots that will keep your feet dry, warm, and protected from injury.

The uppers should be made of watertight material to help keep moisture out; a single-piece upper is more waterproof and durable than one with seams. High boots with stiff ankle support will help keep your ankles from twisting on uneven surfaces. A steel shank in the mid-sole protects your foot from nails, splintered branches, sharp rocks, and other protrusions.

Hiking shoes and light hiking boots have limited support and are intended for walking on smooth, well-maintained trails and carrying a light backpack with only minimal supplies. Mid-weight boots are intended for primitive trails and undemanding off-trail hiking. Off-trail or heavy boots are intended for rough terrain and carrying a heavy backpack containing several days' supplies. The lighter the boot, the easier it is to walk, but you must wear boots that provide the support you need for the conditions.

Boots should be treated periodically with a sealant to keep them waterproof, using a product that is appropriate for the material of the upper.

Crampons attach to boots to provide traction on snow and ice. Hinged crampons flex at the instep and are preferred for most types of mountaineering. Rigid crampons are preferred for climbing steep inclines.

Other specialty footwear that you may want to include in your survival kit:

♦ Waterproof hip boots to keep you dry in thigh-deep water

♦ Water shoes or river boots that are not intended to keep your feet dry, but to protect your feet from sharp rocks or coral

♦ Snowshoes that provide flotation by distributing your weight over a large area so that your feet don't sink into the snow

Wear new shoes or boots doing your normal activities to break them in before packing them with your emergency supplies.

BEDDING & TOWELS

For evacuation, you'll need to take bedding with you, unless you know for certain that you'll be going to a place that provides beds.

Sleeping bags come in various shapes and sizes and are rated by temperature ranges for warm weather, cool weather, cold weather, and extremely cold weather. A four-season bag will provide the most versatility.

If you don't have sleeping bags, you can make your own bedrolls by simply laying out sheets and blankets, rolling them together, and binding both ends of the roll with cord.

If you must sleep outside, it's important not to sleep directly on the ground so you don't lose body heat. To provide insulation from the ground, you can use a foam pad with a down pillow or an air mattress with air pillow. Other alternatives are a folding cot or hammock.

Towels made of microfiber fabric are lightweight, compact, absorbent, and fast-drying. Look for camping towels with a hanging loop for easy drying.

BACKPACKS

Backpacks are an easy way to carry gear while walking. The backpack that you choose should be designed so that the load is carried high and close to your body to reduce the strain on your neck, shoulders, and back. Choose a pack with a brightly colored interior so items are easier to see. Also look for a pack that has straps to hang tools.

Pack individual items in plastic bags to keep them dry. Pack items so that you have easy access to them; for example, make it easy to pull a jacket out of the top instead of having to dump the entire pack to find it in the bottom.

SHELTER

A tent provides portable shelter and requires no fuel to operate. Consider the following characteristics:

- ◆ Sized to accommodate you and your group members
- ◆ Weather-appropriate, either 3-season or 4-season
- ◆ Lightweight
- ◆ Moisture-resistant
- ◆ Windows (allow you to see what's going on outside, and provide cross-ventilation in hot weather)
- ◆ Free-standing design that doesn't require stakes (mighty handy if you're trying to pitch a tent on rock or in loose sand)
- ◆ Interior pockets and loops for storage of gear
- ◆ Color
  - bright color attracts attention and allows you to be easily found (good in a snowstorm, bad for hiding from enemies)
  - muted color allows you to easily hide (good for being inconspicuous, bad if you're lost and want to be found)

Instead of carrying a tent, you can carry a waterproof tarp or plastic sheeting for covering a makeshift frame of tree branches or other plant stalks. Include fasteners such as rawhide strings, wire, cord, or plastic zip ties.

Other pre-fabricated shelters include canopies, portable garages, portable greenhouses, portable sheds, and portable animal shelters.

A motorhome or camper can provide shelter as well as transportation, but you must stockpile enough motor fuel to carry you away from the disaster, and enough propane or other fuel to sustain cooking, heating, and cooling.

MONEY

Stash some cash. In the event of a widespread power outage or the crash of the financial system, your debit cards, credit cards, and ATM cards will be useless.

How much cash is a matter of what your personal comfort zone is. For minor emergencies, a few hundred dollars should be enough. For major emergencies, you might feel better having several thousand at your disposal. In an apocalyptic event, it won't matter how much cash you have, because it will become virtually worthless; survivors will revert to a barter economy.

Stockpile gold. Gold has been the most sought-after precious metal since the beginning of recorded history. If times become desperate, other commodities will be more valuable than gold (such as food and medicine), but a market for gold will always exist. So buy yourself some bling, enjoy wearing it, and be prepared to use it as "money" if the need arises.

PETS

For sheltering-in-place at home with your pets, stock supplies for them just as you will other family members. Include water, food, medications, sanitation supplies, and toys.

Prepare for the situation in which you must shelter-in-place away from home and you cannot reach your pets. Leave keys with your neighbors and ask them to feed your pets in an emergency until you can return home.

Prepare for the situation in which neither you nor your neighbors can care for your pets. Place signage on your house, barn, or other structures to alert others that you have animals on your property.

Microchip your pets. If they become separated from you, you have a better chance of recovering them if they have identification implants. Carry photos of your pets with you.

Keep your pet's shots and identification tags up to date. Your pet's evacuation kit should include medical records, food, water, and medications.

Service animals that help disabled people are allowed in public shelters, but pets are not. If you plan to evacuate to a public shelter, you will have to leave your pets behind or make other arrangements for them.

You can ask friends or relatives if they would be willing to shelter your pets temporarily during an emergency, but in the case of a widespread disaster, they're going to be in the same situation you are, so this is not likely to be a viable option.

Make a list of veterinarians and boarding facilities that could shelter your pets temporarily during an emergency. You can also ask local animal shelters if they provide temporary emergency housing. However, in the case of a widespread disaster, it may not be safe for your pets to stay in the area, and even if it is safe, these facilities may quickly become overwhelmed with animals. Therefore, these facilities may not be viable options.

If you plan to keep your pets with you, be prepared to seek shelter on your own. Make a list of hotels that accept pets. Include local lodgings as well as those within a day's drive of your home.

Water & Purification Supplies

_____ bottled water
_____ filter cartridges
_____ germicidal UV radiation lamp
_____ PET bottles
_____ iodine (liquid, tablets, or crystals)
_____ chlorine (liquid or tablets)
_____ distillation kit
_____ portable osmosis pouches

Food

_____ powdered and/or canned milk
_____ jerky
_____ canned meats (beef, ham, chicken, turkey, tuna, salmon, etc.)
_____ dried and/or canned fruit
_____ dried potatoes, canned vegetables
_____ dried and/or canned beans
_____ canned stew, canned chili
_____ protein bars, energy bars, granola bars
_____ trail mix, nuts, rice cakes
_____ crackers, cheese crackers, peanut butter crackers
_____ ready-to-eat servings of pudding, gelatin, fruit, applesauce, etc.
_____ ready-to-eat soup, condensed canned soup, dried soup mix
_____ canned broth, bouillon cubes
_____ cereal
_____ jam, jelly, preserves, honey, peanut butter
_____ canned and bottled juices, powdered drink mix (cocoa, cider, lemonade)
_____ coffee, tea
_____ MRE's (Meals, Ready-to-Eat) or other self-contained meals
_____ rice, pasta, flour, corn meal
_____ sugar or other sweeteners
_____ vegetable oil
_____ baking powder, baking soda, cornstarch, dry yeast
_____ vinegar
_____ seasonings, flavorings, condiments
_____ hard candies
_____ vitamins, minerals, & other dietary supplements
_____ baby formula, baby food
_____ other special food to meet specific dietary needs

Sanitation

_____ toilet paper
_____ paper towels
_____ facial tissues
_____ feminine hygiene supplies
_____ incontinence supplies
_____ diapers, wipes, & ointment
_____ antibacterial soap
_____ waterless hand sanitizer
_____ pre-moistened wipes
_____ shampoo
_____ toothbrush
_____ toothpaste
_____ floss
_____ mouthwash
_____ deodorant
_____ shaving cream & razors
_____ liquid dish detergent
_____ liquid clothes detergent
_____ chlorine bleach
_____ vinegar
_____ ammonia
_____ hydrogen peroxide
_____ bucket
_____ mop
_____ broom
_____ sponges
_____ dish cloths, dish towels
_____ bath towels
_____ clothes pins & clothes line, drying rack
_____ HEPA (high-efficiency particle arresting) filters for ventilation systems
_____ HEPA (high-efficiency particle arresting) filters for vacuum cleaners
_____ mouse traps & rat traps
_____ insect traps
_____ flypaper
_____ insecticide
_____ plastic bags (snack, sandwich, quart, gallon, 2-gallon, 10-gallon, 30-gallon)
_____ hose
_____ portable hot water heater with fuel, solar shower
_____ portable toilet with chemicals or biodegradable bags

Medical Supplies/First Aid Kit

_____ maintenance medications (insulin, heart medicine, etc.)
_____ insect repellent
_____ sunscreen
_____ electrolyte drinks (for rehydration in case of vomiting and/or diarrhea)
_____ emergency blanket (for treating hypothermia)
_____ cooling vest (for treating heat stroke)
_____ antibacterial soap, antibacterial wipes
_____ antiseptics (alcohol, hydrogen peroxide, iodine, etc.)
_____ triple antibiotic ointment
_____ assorted sterile adhesive bandages
_____ butterfly bandages
_____ sterile gauze pads & roll bandages
_____ triangular bandages
_____ elastic bandages
_____ tourniquet
_____ instant cold packs & instant hot packs
_____ adhesive tape
_____ safety pins
_____ scissors
_____ tweezers
_____ needle & suturing thread
_____ cotton swabs, cotton balls
_____ disposable exam gloves
_____ surgical face masks
_____ CPR masks
_____ thermometer
_____ blood pressure cuff
_____ tongue depressors
_____ medicine dropper
_____ petroleum jelly
_____ saline solution
_____ pain relievers (aspirin, acetaminophen, ibuprofen)
_____ activated charcoal (to counteract poison, only if instructed by medical personnel)
_____ chelating agent such as EDTA (for treating mercury or lead poisoning)
_____ potassium iodide (to treat exposure to radiation)
_____ epinephrine auto-injector (to treat anaphylactic shock from allergic reaction)
_____ antacid (for upset stomach)
_____ anti-emetics (anti-nausea medication for motion sickness)
_____ laxative (for constipation) & anti-diarrheal (for diarrhea)
_____ antihistamines (to treat runny nose & watery eyes)
_____ first-aid manual

Headgear/Eye Wear/Ear Wear/Masks

_____ rain hat
_____ ski mask, stocking hat, cap with flaps, wide-brimmed vented hat
_____ large bandana, neck scarf
_____ sweatband
_____ sunglasses
_____ goggles
_____ thermal earmuffs
_____ dust masks or respiratory masks
_____ snorkel mask

Jackets, Vests, Shirts, Pants

_____ rain suit, slicker, or poncho
_____ jacket or waterproof shell with zip-out lining
_____ battery-heated jackets, vests, & pants
_____ specialty vests (cooling vest, tactical vest)
_____ cargo pants, pants with zip-off legs, brush pants, lined pants
_____ compression shirts & pants
_____ thermal underwear, leggings, or leg warmers

Gloves

_____ leather or cotton work gloves, lined or unlined
_____ battery-heated gloves
_____ gloves with reinforced palms, mesh fabric, long cuffs, or open fingers
_____ gloves with magnetized fingertips for picking up hardware
_____ heat-resistant, puncture-resistant, or cut-resistant gloves
_____ rubber safety gloves for working around electricity

Socks & Footwear

_____ sock liners & hiking socks (lightweight, mid-weight, or heavyweight)
_____ battery-heated socks
_____ compression socks
_____ non-skid socks
_____ flame-resistant socks
_____ hiking shoes or boots
_____ waders or other waterproof boots
_____ water shoes, reef shoes
_____ snowshoes
_____ crampons for boots

Before Disaster

Bedding & Towels

_____ sleeping bag or bed roll
_____ sheets & blankets
_____ pillows
_____ foam pad or mattress
_____ air mattress & pillow with pump
_____ folding cot
_____ hammock
_____ bath towels, hand towels, wash cloths

Shelter

_____ tent
_____ bivouac sack
_____ tarp with cordage & zip ties or portable canopy
_____ mosquito netting

Pets

_____ water
_____ food & manual can opener (if needed)
_____ food & water bowls or bottles
_____ medications
_____ sanitation supplies (litter box, liners, litter, newspapers)
_____ toys & treats
_____ collar, leash, harness, with ID tag, rabies tag, & license
_____ bed, blanket
_____ carrier, cage, or crate
_____ first-aid manual for pets, medical records

Personal Items

_____ items for people with special needs (children, elderly, disabled)
_____ eyeglasses and/or contact lenses & maintenance supplies
_____ hearing aids & extra batteries
_____ canes, walkers, wheelchairs
_____ hand & body lotion
_____ activities (board games, cards, puzzles, books, crafts, needlework)
_____ needle & thread, scissors
_____ pens, pencils, notebooks
_____ wind-up clock
_____ multi-tool
_____ money: cash (paper & coins), debit cards, credit cards

Supplies For Vehicle

_____ bottled water
_____ metal container with matches or lighter (to melt snow for water)
_____ protein bars, granola bars, energy bars
_____ dried fruit
_____ fruit cups, pudding cups
_____ cheese crackers, peanut butter crackers
_____ jerky
_____ MRE's (Meals, Ready-to-Eat)
_____ wet wipes
_____ paper towels
_____ maintenance medications (insulin, blood pressure medication, etc.)
_____ basic first aid kit & manual
_____ hand-cranked AM-FM radio, or battery-powered with extra batteries
_____ CB radio
_____ flashlight & extra batteries
_____ GPS (global positioning system)
_____ maps, atlas
_____ compass
_____ cell phone cable for vehicle port
_____ basic tool kit
_____ battery booster cables
_____ windshield scraper
_____ folding shovel
_____ sand or cat litter
_____ spare tire or tire repair kit & pump
_____ lug wrench
_____ tire chains
_____ tow rope
_____ siphoning hose
_____ emergency triangle
_____ flares
_____ banner or flag for signaling help
_____ sleeping bag or blanket & pillow
_____ extra clothes, appropriate for season
_____ boots or sturdy shoes

Chapter 5

Tools & Equipment

Consider not just the assets but also the liabilities of the equipment and tools that you acquire for survival. As you consider each purchase, think about the following:

▶ **Functionality** - What kind of equipment are you willing to buy? Power tools are great labor-saving devices, but if they run out of fuel or malfunction, they become less valuable than hand tools. A tool with multiple uses can increase your effectiveness in performing tasks. For example, a pickaxe provides two tools on one handle. A screwdriver with multiple tips stored in the handle can replace several separate screwdrivers. A pair of linesman's pliers provides both pliers and a wire-cutting tool in one.

▶ **Physical Capacity** - Are you and other members of your group physically capable of operating the equipment? Can it be adapted to your height, your strength, or other physical limitations?

▶ **Training** - How much training will you need to use tools and equipment that you are unfamiliar with? Can you learn it on your own, or will someone have to teach you? Do you have time for the training? Do you have time to practice with the tool or piece of equipment on a regular basis?

▶ **Durability & Obsolescence** - How long can you expect a piece of equipment to last? Does it have moving parts that will wear down and break? Does it have metal parts that will rust? Does it have belts or seals that will rot? How soon will it become obsolete? Bear in mind that it is often beneficial to wait before buying new technology, as later versions of a product usually have improvements and refinements, sometimes at a cheaper price. Weigh the cost of replacing with the latest version versus keeping the old but sacrificing efficiency or effectiveness.

▶ **Maintenance & Repairs** - Do you know how to maintain it? Do you have time to maintain it? Do you know how to repair it? Are you likely to find the parts to repair it? If manufactured replacement parts become scarce, would they be easy to fabricate, either by you or someone else? As a general rule, don't buy any piece of equipment that you can't maintain and repair. Either know how to maintain and repair it yourself, or have enough money to pay someone else to maintain and repair it, assuming that someone with the required expertise will be available when needed. Otherwise the equipment will become useless to you.

▶ **Logistics** - Think about the size, shape, and weight of each item. Do you have room to store it? Can it be disassembled for storage? If relocating becomes necessary, how much will it cost in time, money, and energy to move it? Are suitable alternatives available? For example, if you want to include gear for water travel among your survival equipment, an inflatable raft would make more sense than a canoe because a canoe is heavy and bulky.

▶ **Redundancy** - Give yourself as many options as possible. Buy a variety of tools that can alternate for one another in case your intended tool fails. For example, a crosscut saw and a hacksaw are designed for different purposes, but in an emergency, one could substitute for the other. To increase your redundancy even more, if you have the money and storage space, stock up on duplicate equipment. Duplicates are useful to have as backups, to disassemble for spare parts, and to use for bartering.

The topics in this chapter include:

- energy sources & equipment
    - lighting
    - heating
    - cooking
    - cooling
    - refrigeration
- communications equipment & services
- vehicles

ENERGY

You will need energy in some form for lighting, heating, cooking, cooling, refrigeration, and operating appliances, equipment, and power tools.

Fuel comes in many forms: candle wax, animal dung, wood, coal, gasoline, diesel, kerosene, natural gas, propane, butane, alcohol, biofuels, batteries, etc.

You can buy equipment that uses various sources of energy, such as light produced by burning fuel with an open flame or light produced by a chemical reaction. Some individual pieces of equipment can use more than one source of energy, such as corded appliances that can also use batteries, or lanterns that can use more than one kind of liquid fuel.

The value of energy depends on your needs and budget. For example, if you need to refrigerate medications or operate life-sustaining equipment, your need is relatively high and energy will be a high priority for you in an emergency situation. Or if you live in extreme heat or extreme cold, your need is higher than someone who lives in a more moderate climate.

The pages at the end of the chapter list some alternate tools and alternate sources of energy. Some are low-tech, some are high-tech. Some are short-term and some are long-term. Some are intended only as backups for use during temporary power outages, while others can offer a solution to get you off the grid permanently. Some are heavy-duty and suitable for sheltering-in-place, while others are portable and better suited to evacuation.

☠ **Warning: To avoid carbon monoxide poisoning, never use gas-powered equipment in an attached garage or closed living space. Generators, portable grills, space heaters, or any other equipment or appliances powered by any kind of gas must be vented to the outside.**

☠ **Warning: If you will be using a portable generator, be prepared to turn off the main breaker in your home's electrical panel to prevent backfeed.**

☠ **Warning: Do not vent a solid-fuel appliance into a chimney that is used by a gas furnace or gas water heater. This is dangerous.**

Lighting

You have a variety of lighting choices:

- long-burning emergency candle with butane lighter or waterproof matches in a waterproof container; if you plan to use candles for light, think about where you'll put them to keep them lit and not create a hazard; open flames should not be used in windy conditions

- oil lamp with matches, wicks, and fuel (kerosene, lamp oil, etc.)

- lantern with matches, mantles, and fuel (propane, kerosene, butane, etc.)

- flare

- glow stick/light stick

- battery-powered flashlight with batteries and charger

- solar-powered flashlight

- hand-cranked/windup flashlight

- rechargeable wall-socket-mounted flashlight; it stays charged and turns on automatically when the power goes out; put one in each bedroom and throughout the house to illuminate the way out at night

- headlamp with batteries - mounted on your forehead, this leaves your hands free to steady your way or carry other objects

- work light - electric light mounted on a stand or hanging from a hook that allows you to aim the beam of light at your task

- strobe light, to discourage intruders or to alert rescue workers of your location

- solar-powered torch

- torch with matches, wicks, and fuel (propane, lamp oil, etc.)

"Strike-anywhere" matches can be lit by striking them against any surface with friction. "Storm" matches are coated with wax to make them waterproof and a combustible compound to make them burn even in heavy winds.

Keep on hand fuel, matches, wicks, mantles, batteries, and bulbs.

Heating

If you heat your home with electric or natural gas, here are some other options for staying warm during an outage:

- wood-burning or coal-fired central furnace with plenty of wood or coal; without electricity, the blower won't work, but heat will naturally radiate upwards even without a fan

- free-standing stove with fuel (wood, coal, fuel oil)

- portable space heater with fuel (propane, kerosene)

- fire pit with wood to burn

- smudge pot with fuel; for use outdoors to help protect crops against frost

Cooking

If you have an electric or gas range, here are some other options for cooking during an outage:

- canned fuel (jellied alcohol) for use underneath cans or pots

- wood-burning stove with wood to burn

- camp stove with fuel (propane, butane, gasoline)

- solar cooker – you can buy one ready-made, or make your own by wrapping aluminum foil over cardboard

- portable grill with fuel (propane, charcoal)

- hibachi with charcoal

- fire pit with wood to burn

- battery-powered microwave oven

Here are utensils and equipment that may be helpful:

- a grill or grate with legs tall enough to sit over a container of canned fuel or a bed of coals

- skewers or a long-handled fork

- pots with legs or pots with handles and a tripod to set over a fire

Use cooking fuel efficiently:

♦ Using a lid increases the efficiency of your cookware and therefore consumes less fuel.

♦ Use the pot size that matches your quantity of food. Using a large pot to cook a small quantity of food wastes fuel.

♦ Combine several foods such as meat, vegetables, and pasta to cook in one pot. Cooking in one large pot uses fuel more efficiently than cooking in several small pots.

♦ Wide shallow pots cook more efficiently than tall narrow pots.

♦ The material makes a difference:

  * Copper is the most efficient heat conductor of any metal for cooking.

  * Aluminum is an excellent heat conductor and is very fuel-efficient for cooking.

  * Cast iron heats and cools slowly; it retains heat well and is fuel-efficient for cooking food that has a long cooking time.

  * Carbon steel heats and cools quickly; it requires relatively little fuel to cook food that has a short cooking time.

  * Stainless steel does not conduct heat well compared to other metals. Stainless steel that is clad in copper or aluminum ensures heat will be distributed more evenly.

  * Glass and ceramic are the least fuel-efficient types of cookware.

Cooling

In extremely high temperatures, it is critical to keep the body from overheating, especially for infants, the elderly, and those with medical conditions. If you lose power and don't have access to air conditioning or corded electric fans, here are some alternatives:

- ◆ battery-powered fan with batteries and charger

- ◆ battery-powered misting fan with batteries and charger

- ◆ evaporative cooler (also called a swamp cooler, desert cooler, or wet-air cooler)

- ◆ rigid or folding hand fans made of paper, fabric, or feathers

Refrigeration

If you lose power for more than 24 hours, the food in your refrigerator will start to spoil, and the food in your freezer will start to thaw. Use one or more of these as a backup:

- ◆ insulated cooler with ice packs or gel packs

- ◆ portable refrigerator that runs on a 12-volt vehicle battery

- ◆ battery-powered refrigerator

- ◆ solar-powered refrigerator

Operating Appliances, Equipment, & Power Tools

In the event of a power outage, you can rely on battery-powered devices, provided that you have a stockpile of batteries. The initial cost of rechargeable batteries is higher than one-time use batteries, but reusing them several times will make them cheaper in the long run. Keep rechargeable batteries charged so they will be useful in case of a power outage. Keep one-time use batteries on hand in case the power outage lasts longer than the charge on the rechargeable batteries. Keep both rechargeable batteries and one-time use batteries in various sizes (AAA, AA, C, D, etc.)

As an alternative to relying on batteries, you can install a standby generator in your home. This is a stationary unit that runs on gas or propane and is hard-wired into your home's electrical system to provide power if your electricity from the grid goes out. Since it is dependent on another fuel source, it will provide electricity only as long as it has fuel.

More common is a portable gasoline- or diesel-powered generator. It is an excellent backup for operating electrical devices and recharging batteries when electrical power goes out. This is especially important if you use well water and need electricity to operate the pump. Remember to stockpile fuel to run the generator, and test it periodically to make sure it starts. Be prepared to lock and tag the main circuit breaker on your home's electrical panel to prevent backfeed. Install an interlock or transfer switch to allow your electrical panel to feed off the generator; otherwise, you will need several extension cords to run from the generator to the various appliances in your home.

A high-tech solution is to install "green" technology, such as solar shingles, solar panels, or a wind turbine to generate your own electricity and become independent of the power grid.

COMMUNICATIONS EQUIPMENT & SERVICES

During a disaster, you need news, advisories, and other information. You need to stay in touch with the other members of your group, to let them know your location and your condition. You need the capabilities to both receive and send information.

Have a variety of communications devices available. The more ways you have to communicate, the more likely you will be able to connect with others in an emergency.

Communications devices require some kind of power source: a wire plugged into an outlet of a building or vehicle, a portable battery, a solar cell, or a hand crank. Corded TV's, radios, and computers are convenient for everyday home use, but they won't help you during a power outage. Battery-powered devices are a good substitute during power outages, but they are only for short-term use, until the battery loses power. Solar-powered devices provide easily renewable energy. Wind-up devices only require you to have the ability to turn the crank.

A gas- or diesel-powered generator can be used to operate corded devices during a power outage, or to recharge batteries. Solar chargers can recharge a variety of devices, as long as you have access to the sun.

Assess your risks and your resources. Are you in a remote area? Are you likely to encounter severe weather? How much money do you have to devote to communication products and services?

Consolidate whenever possible. Buy a combination radio with AM/FM/NOAA. (NOAA is the National Oceanic and Atmospheric Administration. These are the folks who operate the National Weather Service and broadcast weather advisories, watches, and warnings.) Buy devices that offer more than one power option, such as corded and battery-powered, or battery-powered and hand-cranked.

For devices that are battery-powered only, remember to keep your batteries charged, and have spares on hand.

Other devices that can be used for signaling include whistles, flashlights, and mirrors.

- wire-based phone - Keep a land line at home. This phone will work even when your electricity is out, unless a catastrophe strikes your phone service carrier or knocks out the transmission lines. Cell phones may be useless during an emergency if a spike in call volume overloads the network or a tower is damaged.

- cordless phones - Keep cordless phones throughout the house so you are always near a means to communicate in an emergency, and you can carry the handset with you from room to room.

- cell phone with text messaging service, extra battery, and wind-up charger - Subscribe to text messaging with your cell phone. Even if a call won't go through during an emergency, a text message might, as it requires less bandwidth.

- satellite phone with a solar charger - Both the hardware and subscription service are expensive, but this is the device of choice in remote locations where cell-phone service is unavailable. If satellites are knocked out, these phones won't work, but this is unlikely.

- wire-based computer with internet service & email account

- battery-powered computer

- battery-powered TV

- battery-powered or hand-cranked/wind-up AM/FM radio

- battery-powered or hand-cranked/wind-up NOAA weather radio - You can leave it on 24/7 to receive alerts whenever the National Weather Service issues a storm warning. Get one with SAME (Specific Area Message Encoding) technology to limit the alerts to your immediate vicinity.

- walkie-talkies or handie-talkies

- battery-powered citizens' band (CB) radio

- amateur (ham) radio

- marine VHF radio

- soup cans & string (fun for the kids!)

VEHICLES

For your evacuation plan, have a primary means of transportation as well as several alternates. You may have a choice of going by land, water, or air, using either private or public transportation.

If public transportation is available, know how to get to the terminals or stops, and learn when the first and last departures are. Teach your children how to read a bus schedule, how to buy a token, and how to get a transfer.

During an evacuation from a large urban area, roads usually become choked with traffic, so traveling on foot may actually take you away from the area faster. Being "on foot" doesn't mean you have to walk; skates can allow you to cover more ground; however, they aren't suitable for rough terrain. If you're caught in a heavy snowfall, cross-country skis or snowshoes may be the best option.

You may think of a nearby river only in recreational terms, but for hundreds of years before you got here, the natives used it for transportation, and it can, in fact, carry you far, far away.

Modern life rafts are typically equipped with a survival pack tethered to the floor of the raft. Included are food rations, water pouches, medical supplies, signaling devices, a fishing kit, and other survival gear. The canopy may have a device for catching rain water. The raft may have water-activated batteries that automatically turn on a flashing light so you can see where you're going if you must abandon ship at night. To become familiar with how life rafts work, schedule a visit to a marina and watch the inspection of a life raft.

When you think of traveling by plane, you may only think of buying a ticket on a big commercial airliner. But thousands of county and municipal airports across the country support general aviation, and you might be able to rent a plane with a pilot. You might also be able to hitch a ride on a military transport.

Land

♦ automobile or truck
♦ bicycle
♦ moped, scooter, or motorcycle
♦ golf cart
♦ all-terrain vehicle
♦ roller skates
♦ ice skates
♦ snow skis
♦ snowshoes
♦ snowmobile
♦ dogsled
♦ draft animals: horses, mules, donkeys, etc.
♦ taxi
♦ streetcar, trolley, or cable car
♦ bus, local or long-distance, or school bus
♦ train, commuter or long-distance

Water

♦ kayak
♦ rowboat
♦ canoe
♦ raft
♦ sailboat
♦ power boat
♦ personal watercraft
♦ water taxi
♦ ferry
♦ barge
♦ ocean-going ships: cruise, fishing, freighter

Air

♦ airplane
♦ ultralight
♦ seaplane
♦ helicopter
♦ hot air balloon
♦ dirigible

Before Disaster

Lighting

_____ emergency candles with lighter or matches in a waterproof container
_____ oil lamp with matches, wicks, and fuel (kerosene, lamp oil, etc.)
_____ lantern with matches, mantles, and fuel (propane, kerosene, butane, etc.)
_____ flare
_____ glow stick/light stick
_____ battery-powered flashlight with batteries and charger
_____ solar-powered flashlight
_____ hand-cranked/windup flashlight
_____ rechargeable wall-socket-mounted flashlight
_____ headlamp with batteries
_____ work light
_____ hanging work light with cage around bulb to protect it from breakage
_____ strobe light
_____ solar-powered torch
_____ torch with matches, wicks, and fuel (propane, lamp oil, etc.)

Heating

_____ wood-burning or coal-fired central furnace with wood or coal
_____ free-standing stove with fuel (wood, coal, fuel oil)
_____ portable space heater with fuel (propane, kerosene)
_____ fire pit with wood to burn
_____ smudge pot with fuel (for outdoor use)

Cooking

_____ canned fuel (jellied alcohol) for use underneath cans or pots
_____ wood-burning stove with wood to burn
_____ camp stove with fuel (propane, butane, gasoline)
_____ solar cooker
_____ portable grill with fuel (propane, charcoal) or hibachi with charcoal
_____ fire pit with wood to burn
_____ a grill or grate with tall legs
_____ skewers or a long-handled fork, coffee pot & filters
_____ pots with legs, pots with handles and a tripod, lids for pots
_____ knives, cutting board, ladle, measuring cups & spoons, tongs
_____ thermometer, timer, rolling pin, grater, funnel, spatula, potholders
_____ manual can opener, whisk, strainer, & other assorted utensils
_____ plates, bowls, cups, flatware

Cooling

_____ battery-powered fan with batteries and charger
_____ battery-powered misting fan with batteries and charger
_____ evaporative cooler (also called a swamp cooler, desert cooler, or wet-air cooler)
_____ rigid or folding hand fans made of paper, fabric, or feathers

Refrigeration

_____ insulated cooler with ice packs or gel packs
_____ portable refrigerator that runs on a 12-volt vehicle battery
_____ battery-powered refrigerator
_____ solar-powered refrigerator

Operating Appliances, Equipment, & Power Tools

_____ batteries, both one-time use and rechargeable, in various sizes
_____ standby generator hard-wired into house & fuel
_____ portable gasoline- or diesel-powered generator & fuel
_____ solar shingles
_____ solar panels
_____ wind turbine

Communications Equipment & Services

_____ wire-based phone
_____ cordless phone
_____ cell phone with text messaging service, extra battery, and wind-up charger
_____ satellite phone with a solar charger
_____ wire-based computer with internet service & email account
_____ battery-powered computer
_____ battery-powered TV
_____ battery-powered or hand-cranked/wind-up AM/FM radio
_____ battery-powered or hand-cranked/wind-up NOAA weather radio
_____ walkie-talkies or handie-talkies
_____ battery-powered citizens' band (CB) radio
_____ amateur (ham) radio
_____ marine VHF radio
_____ whistle
_____ flashlight or mirror
_____ soup cans & string (fun for the kids!)

Miscellaneous Tools & Equipment (both manual & powered)

_____ hammers
_____ screwdrivers (flathead & crosshead)
_____ wrenches
_____ sockets
_____ pliers
_____ clamps, vises
_____ chisel
_____ pry bar
_____ file or rasp, sander
_____ plane
_____ wire stripper, crimper, & cutter
_____ utility knife, box cutter, bolt cutter, shears, scissors
_____ saws
_____ miter box
_____ tape measure
_____ square
_____ level
_____ punches
_____ drill
_____ pick ax or hatchet
_____ shovel
_____ sickle, scythe, machete
_____ rake
_____ hoe
_____ fork
_____ wheelbarrow
_____ air compressor
_____ welder with tanks
_____ hardware (nuts, bolts, screws, nails, etc.)
_____ fire extinguisher (ABC type)
_____ duct tape
_____ extension cords
_____ hunting knife

Personal Protection Equipment

_____ hardhat with safety visor or shield
_____ welding helmet or goggles, welding jacket
_____ safety glasses, smoke-escape hood
_____ earplugs, acoustic ear muffs
_____ work gloves

Chapter 6

Personal Practices

This chapter is about steps you can take to help minimize your exposure to catastrophic events.

The topics in this chapter include:
- health
- vaccination
- hygiene
- travel & transportation
- weather
- suspicious activities
- hijacking or other hostage situation
- terrorist targets
- business owner
- financial collapse
- basic skills

HEALTH

Get in shape and keep yourself in top physical condition with proper nutrition, exercise, and sleep. For your exercise regimen, include aerobic exercises (such as walking, running, or cycling) to increase cardiovascular endurance, anaerobic exercises (such as weightlifting) to build muscle strength, and flexibility exercises (such as stretching) to improve the range of motion of muscles and joints. Being healthy and fit will help your body fight infections, will make it easier to evacuate on foot, if you need to, and will allow you to better tolerate reduced rations, if you need to.

Stay emotionally fit. Simplify your existence, reduce the stress in your life, and keep a positive attitude.

VACCINATION

If a contagion threatens to spread and an epidemic or a pandemic is predicted, you must decide whether to be vaccinated, assuming a vaccine is available. If you have children, you must also decide whether to vaccinate them against the contagion, as well as a variety of typical childhood diseases such as polio, chickenpox, and measles. Children and adults with robust immune systems are better able to tolerate catastrophic events. Those with immune systems weakened by disease are more susceptible to additional infections.

If you will be traveling outside of the U.S., you may be exposed to diseases that are uncommon in America, and you must decide whether to be vaccinated. Check the websites for the U. S. State Department, the Centers for Disease Control, and the World Health Organization for travel advisories and advice on vaccinations for the areas you will be visiting. Check well in advance, as some vaccines require significant advance notice to obtain.

Vaccines may have caused irreparable damage in rare cases, but they have undoubtedly saved millions of lives.

When considering vaccination, be sure you understand what it can be expected to do for you:

- A vaccine immunizes against one or more strains of a microorganism. It does nothing to protect you from other strains of the pathogen that aren't included in the vaccine, and pathogens continuously mutate.

- A vaccine does not provide immediate immunity. It may take several days or weeks for your body to produce the antibodies that provide protection against the disease.

- A vaccine may not provide full immunity. You may still contract the disease, although it would likely be a mild case.

- A vaccine may not provide permanent immunity.

No vaccine is 100% safe. But the medical establishment maintains that the probability of an adverse reaction to the vaccine is smaller than the probability of complications or death from the disease. To make an informed decision, find out:

♦ the side effects of the vaccine

♦ the percentage of people who are permanently disabled by the vaccine

♦ the percentage of people who die from the vaccine

♦ the symptoms of the disease

♦ the percentage of people who are permanently disabled by the disease

♦ the percentage of people who die from the disease

The decision to vaccinate or not should be made only after careful consideration of all available facts. Research the pro's and con's, and decide for yourself.

No one can force you to be vaccinated against your will. However, if you decline vaccination, you may face certain restrictions, such as not being allowed to participate in certain activities or not being allowed to travel to certain places.

HYGIENE

Make personal hygiene a priority to minimize your exposure to bacteria and viruses. You won't know an epidemic is developing until a lot of other people have already become sick. The best way to avoid becoming a victim in an epidemic or pandemic is to maintain optimal health and to observe excellent personal hygiene.

♦ Wash your hands frequently. Wash after being outside and in public, always after using the bathroom, always before preparing food, and always before eating.

♦ Wash your hands with soap and hot running water. It's not necessary to use antibacterial soap on a regular basis, but it may be a good idea if your immune system is suppressed. Lather well, and scrub between your fingers, under your fingernails, and over the backs of your hands up to your wrists. Teach your children to take at least enough time to sing the ABC's all the way through. Rinse well.

♦ Carry antibacterial wipes or waterless sanitizer with you. Use after you've touched surfaces in public, such as door handles, menus, ATM buttons, fuel nozzle handles, shopping carts, money, etc.

♦ Avoid sharing personal items such as razors, toothbrushes, combs, brushes, cosmetic applicators, etc.

♦ Avoid crowds of people and minimize physical contact with strangers. Avoid contact with unfamiliar people, stray dogs and cats, and wild animals that may carry disease.

♦ Wear protective clothing when you perform physical work. A long-sleeved shirt, long pants, boots, and gloves will help protect your body against cuts and scrapes. If you get an abrasion that breaks the skin, allow the wound to bleed enough to clean it out and then apply first aid.

♦ Wear a mask. If you work in a position where you come in frequent contact with the general public, wear a mask. This is especially important if you have a weakened immune system, if you come in contact with international travelers, and during cold and flu season.

♦ Spray insect repellent on clothes and exposed skin to reduce bites from disease-carrying insects.

Food Handling

♦ Keep kitchen surfaces clean by wiping with disinfectant.

♦ Wash cutting boards and knives after every use. If you cut raw meat or poultry or fish, wash the board and knife before using them with any other food.

♦ Change dishcloths and dishtowels at every meal to retard the growth of germs.

♦ Wash raw food thoroughly before eating.

♦ Heat cooked food thoroughly before eating.

♦ Keep hot foods hot and cold foods cold to retard the growth of bacteria.

♦ To avoid spreading germs, don't double-dip finger food into a common container.

♦ Avoid sharing plates, glasses, eating utensils, or bites of food.

♦ Keep your freezer full, with water-filled jugs if necessary. During a power outage, frozen food will keep from spoiling longer if the freezer is packed full.

Mail Handling

One way to reduce your risk of exposure from contaminated mail is to reduce the amount of paper mail that you open. You can pay bills, balance your checkbook, and shop online. It's personally safer and "greener," too.

For mail that you do have to open:

♦ Wear gloves.

♦ Avoid sniffing letters or packages before opening them.

♦ Open mail slowly with a letter opener.

♦ Wash your hands after handling mail.

♦ If you receive an unexpected letter or package from a stranger, beware of the following:

    ♦ no return address
    ♦ addressed incorrectly
    ♦ misspellings of common words
    ♦ excessive postage
    ♦ foreign postage
    ♦ postmark city/state different from return-address city/state
    ♦ marked "Confidential" or "Do Not X-ray"
    ♦ stains, dirt, or oil on the outside
    ♦ strange odor
    ♦ powder of an unknown origin inside
    ♦ threatening messages inside

♦ If an item is suspicious, seal it in plastic and immediately notify the police or the delivery service.

TRAVEL & TRANSPORTATION

♦ When you travel, let a friend or relative know of your plans. Tell them your destination, your expected time of arrival, and the route you plan to take. If any of your plans change, let them know.

♦ If you are in unfamiliar territory, stay on or close to the main roads so help will be nearby if you need it. Stay away from roads that are lightly traveled. This is especially important in the mountains, where you might get caught in a snowstorm, or crossing a desert.

♦ If you have to take a detour, be on the lookout for signposts to guide your way. When you come to a fork in the road, be sure you take the right path.

♦ If the road has a gate, this usually means it is either a seasonal road or a utility road (such as used for logging or maintenance of power lines). Avoid these roads, since they are not highly traveled and not well maintained.

♦ Reduce your risk of exposure to dangerous situations by conducting business online. Instead of taking a train or plane to travel long-distance to a meeting, use the Internet to have an online meeting.

♦ When you take a trip, make it look like someone is still home. Use timers to turn on a series of lights at different times. Have someone collect your mail, newspapers, advertisements, and packages, or have those deliveries held. Have someone mow the lawn, rake the leaves, or shovel the snow.

♦ When you travel, be inconspicuous. To avoid being a target of crime, don't act like a tourist. Avoid being flashy or loud. Don't wear expensive jewelry and don't carry the latest electronics. If you travel internationally, research the customs and show respect for the culture you are visiting. Avoid wearing clothing with American slogans or logos, or clothing that is distinctly American (i.e., leave your cowboy hat and spurs at home).

♦ Stay in a trusted hotel. Spend a few extra bucks to stay where it's safe.

- Pack a door wedge and use it to hold your hotel-room door closed even if someone breaks the lock.

- Avoid high-crime areas and isolated areas while you are out conducting business or sightseeing.

- Keep track of your wallet and personal belongings. Carry your money and passport in a money belt underneath your clothes to help deter pickpockets.

- Avoid routines. Vary the times that you come and go at your hotel, and vary the routes you take.

- Be aware of your surroundings. Always know what's going on around you and who is in your vicinity. Keep track of where your family members are, especially children. Look around, and let other people see that you are being observant. Project self-confidence.

- Notice if anyone is following you. Use reflections in windows or car mirrors to monitor what's going on behind you. If you think you are being followed, stop at a shop window, cross the street, or turn a corner and observe what happens. If they stay behind you, get to safety. Go into a store or other public place or go to a busy intersection. Do not lead anyone back to your home or hotel.

- Avoid anyone who appears to be loitering. In foreign countries, be wary of locals who approach you. Avoid involvement in arguments or other incidents with the locals.

- If you rent a car in a foreign country, buy insurance. If you are involved in an accident, contact the police. Some locals deliberately become involved in fender-benders with foreigners just to shake them down.

Traveling On Foot

- Travel in pairs or groups.
- Avoid routes that are dark and isolated.
- Carry a canister of pepper spray. (Check the laws in your state regarding restrictions.)
- Carry a whistle to attract attention if someone tries to assault you.
- Carry your purse, briefcase, or other parcels close to your body.
- If you're in an isolated area, especially at night, avoid getting into an elevator alone with a stranger or group of strangers.
- If you are leaving a facility at night, ask the security office to provide you with an escort to your car or bus stop.
- If someone drops you off at home at night, ask them to wait with their headlights on until you are safely inside your home.
- If you have to walk even a few steps from the street to your entrance, be ready with your key so you don't have to fumble around looking for it while standing at your doorstep. Make a fist and carry your key protruding between your fingers so you can poke an attacker, if necessary.
- Beware of tricks. Pedophiles lure children into their vehicles by telling them they need help looking for a lost puppy or kitten, or that their parents have been injured. Teach your children never to go anywhere with strangers. Give your children a secret password that no one would be able to guess, and teach them to require this password from anyone who claims to have instructions from you about what to do in an unfamiliar situation.
- Anytime they need help, children should be taught to approach someone they know they can trust, such as a teacher, a bus driver, a police officer, or a firefighter.
- Locate neighborhood buildings such as restaurants, convenience stores, fire stations, libraries, and city buses that display the yellow diamond-shaped "Safe Place" signs, and teach your children that these are places to go for immediate help and safety.
- Always have at least two routes of escape. Whenever you enter a building, make a mental note of where the exits are. In a multi-story building, locate the stairs.
- When you check into a hotel, take the stairs when you leave your room so you'll become familiar with at least two exits and where you'll come out at the bottom.

Traveling In Vehicles

Private Vehicle

♦ Keep your vehicle in good repair and up-to-date on maintenance in case you need to evacuate without notice.

♦ Keep your vehicle's fuel tank full in case you need to evacuate without notice. Fill up when the fuel gauge drops to half a tank.

♦ When you're standing beside your vehicle filling it with fuel, look for the emergency shut-off for the dispensers in case of fire.

♦ While driving, keep the doors locked and the windows shut.

♦ Be alert when you are stopped at intersections.

♦ Try to stay in control of your movements. Keep enough distance from other vehicles so they can't block you in traffic.

♦ Park in areas that are well lit, with security cameras and patrols.

♦ Park as close to building entrances as possible. Avoid parking in isolated areas.

♦ Avoid parking between vehicles larger than your own to avoid being hidden from view.

♦ Look around before getting out of your vehicle. Avoid areas where people are loitering. Lock the doors when you leave.

♦ When you are ready to return to your vehicle, get your key out of your pocket or purse so you don't have to fumble around looking for it while standing beside your vehicle. Make a fist and carry your key protruding between your fingers so you can poke an attacker, if necessary.

♦ Look around before getting in your vehicle. Make sure no one is hanging around outside the vehicle, and make sure no one is inside your vehicle. As soon as you get in your vehicle, lock the doors and turn on the lights.

Public Transportation

♦ Be aware of the people and activities around you. If you observe suspicious or nervous behavior, alert a crew member.

♦ Be aware of the route being taken so you will always know where you are. In a taxi, make note of the streets you pass. On a bus or train, keep track of the stops you pass. On a ferry, look for landmarks. On a plane, ask what the flight path will be, especially over water.

Bus or Train

♦   If you are waiting at a stop, stand near other passengers. Avoid standing by yourself, where you can be vulnerable to assault.

♦   Once on board, sit near other passengers. Avoid sitting alone.

♦   On a double-decker bus or in a multi-level train car, a seat on the lower level provides quicker access to a door exit.

♦   In a frontal impact on a bus, the front seats will sustain the most damage; in a rear impact, the rear seats will sustain the most damage; in a side impact, the window seats will sustain the most damage. The safest seats are generally the aisle seats in the middle of the bus.

♦   In a head-on collision between two trains, the front cars of both trains will sustain damage. In a front-to-rear collision between two trains, the front train will sustain the most damage to its rear cars, and the rear train will sustain the most damage to its front cars. In a derailment, the window seats will likely sustain the most damage. So try to sit in a middle car, in an aisle seat against the bulkhead. Choose a seat facing the rear so you won't be thrown forward in a crash.

♦   Study the windows so you know how to operate them in an emergency.

Plane

♦   The safest seats on a plane are usually aisle seats near an exit. These seats offer the quickest way out.

♦   Try to book a seat as far as possible from the fuel. Fuel is usually stored in the wings, sometimes in the belly, and occasionally in the tail.

♦   Regardless of where your assigned seat is, locate all of the exits when you board a plane.

Ship

♦   Damage to the hull exposes the lower cabins to flooding. Outer cabins on higher decks offer the quickest escape.

♦   As soon as you board, determine the location of life jackets, lifeboats, and other emergency gear.

WEATHER

Stay Informed about weather conditions such as droughts, flooding, snow storms, and dust storms so you can modify your behavior accordingly.

Droughts lower the levels of groundwater, lakes, and rivers, and may result in water rationing. Reduced rainfall results in low crop yields, leading in turn to increased food prices. Flooding may also reduce crop yields, increasing food prices as well. Staying attuned to these effects can help you adjust your inventory of water, food, and other supplies.

Use your NOAA radio or the Internet to monitor precipitation:

- The Crop Moisture Index assesses short-term dryness and wetness.

- The Palmer Drought Severity Index assesses long-term dryness and wetness.

Blizzards are characterized by winds of at least 35 mph and visibility of less than ¼ mile. Snow, ice, and wind can knock out power lines and make roads impassable.

Dust storms occur in hot, dry, windy conditions. They are characterized by strong violent winds of at least 25 mph, carrying fine particles of sand and clay that reduce visibility to zero. They may rise up to 10,000 feet and spread over hundreds of miles.

Before traveling, listen to local TV or radio broadcasts or use the Internet to check weather conditions. If a thunderstorm, blizzard, or dust storm is predicted, postpone your trip or detour around the storm.

If you participate in snow sports, monitor changes in the conditions that may cause an avalanche.

- ◆ Keep an eye on the weather, temperature, wind direction, and snow-pack conditions. Pay attention to the Avalanche Danger Scale.

- ◆ Use an inclinometer to assess avalanche potential before heading down a slope.

- ◆ Ski or snowmobile in pairs or groups, but go down the slope one at a time so that in case an avalanche occurs, everyone in your group won't be caught in it.

- ◆ Stay away from the edges of a drop-off.

- ◆ Wear an avalanche beacon and set your transceiver to transmit so you can be found if you become buried. Change it to receive if you need to find someone who is lost.

- ◆ Carry a compass to use in case you get disoriented.

- ◆ Carry a collapsible avalanche probe or use probe ski poles.

- ◆ Carry a collapsible shovel.

SUSPICIOUS ACTIVITIES

If you notice someone or something suspicious, move away from the area and report it to the police, security personnel, a utility company, etc. Any of the following situations should raise questions:

♦ A person who is overdressed for the weather (such as wearing a coat in warm temperatures) or is wearing baggy clothes that may be hiding a weapon underneath.

♦ A person who shows an unwarranted interest in the routines of particular individuals or groups, or unusual interest in high-profile targets such as military or other government installations, monuments, etc.; unwarranted interest in security systems or access to restricted areas; unusual interest in the response times of emergency services. Someone taking a photo of the U.S. Capitol isn't suspicious; someone taking a photo of its surveillance system would be.

♦ An unexpected delivery from a stranger.

♦ Out-of-place or strange objects:

  * A briefcase, suitcase, backpack, bag, box, or other container left unattended in a crowd. If you see a suspicious package of any kind, leave it alone. Don't pick it up or open it; move away from it. Notify someone in authority, such as a security guard, a maintenance supervisor, or the police, but do not report it by cell phone or shortwave radio until you are at least 100 yards from it.
  * A vehicle that seems overloaded or is leaking an unidentified substance, especially if the vehicle is parked near a high-profile target such as a government building or an arena that holds lots of people.

♦ The smell of gas or a hissing sound near a gas line. Move away from the area and report it to the gas company or the police.

♦ Remember: "If you see something, say something."

HIJACKING OR OTHER HOSTAGE SITUATION

Large groups of passengers on planes and ships are typically taken hostage because their captors want to make some political statement or they want money to fund their wars or other terrorist activities. Smaller groups of people or an individual may be taken hostage incidental to a robbery, or maybe just because some unstable person is having a meltdown. In all of these scenarios, you will have virtually no warning, so the best way to protect yourself is to minimize the opportunities for such occurrences and to remain aware of your surroundings.

You can try to minimize your chances of being in a politically-motivated hostage situation by avoiding international travel to high-risk destinations.

You can try to minimize your chances of being taken hostage during a robbery by avoiding high-crime areas.

Stay alert to what is going on around you in public. If you see a hostage situation start to unfold, escape if you can.

Avoid cruises to areas where pirates roam the high seas.

If you plan to travel overseas, first check the U. S. State department for travel advisories.

Traveling on your own can make you less noticeable than traveling with a group, but also more easily overcome. On the other hand, traveling with a group of other tourists can make you a bigger target than traveling alone. If you travel with a group, it may be safer to travel with other nationalities, rather than a group of Americans.

Stay informed about local, regional, national, and international events. Read a newspaper, listen to a radio, watch TV, or surf the Internet. Know what's going on in the world around you.

TERRORIST TARGETS

Terrorists pick their targets for the impact they will make. High-profile targets are those that will make a big impact in loss of life, property damage, and/or disruption of services.

Avoid likely targets of an attack, such as large public venues, especially on or near anniversary dates of other attacks, such as 7/7 or 9/11.

♦ mass-transit terminals
♦ passenger trains/subways
♦ planes
♦ cruise ships
♦ ferries
♦ bridges
♦ tunnels
♦ freight trains, especially those hauling hazardous materials
♦ chemical factories and refineries
♦ nuclear power plants
♦ water purification, storage, and pumping facilities
♦ fuel storage depots
♦ food irradiation facilities
♦ bio weapons research labs
♦ military bases
♦ dams
♦ large office buildings, especially federal sites
♦ communication lines and satellite dishes
♦ TV stations
♦ monuments, especially federal sites
♦ resorts
♦ sports stadiums
♦ concert halls
♦ shopping malls
♦ amusement parks

BUSINESS OWNER

Business owners, by their very nature, like to think they're in charge, but the fact is, some forces are beyond their control. Nobody was more surprised to lose their livelihoods than the owners of the GM and Chrysler dealerships who lost their franchises during the bankruptcies of 2009. They weren't "employees," whose employment was subject to the whims of a boss. They were small-business owners who thought they were in control of their own destinies.

Besides financial difficulties, your business operations could be interrupted by an earthquake, a fire, a major power outage, a flood, a hurricane, a tornado, or other catastrophic event. Such a disaster could happen to your own facility, or it could happen to a major supplier, leaving you without raw materials or products to sell, or it could happen to a major customer, leaving you with a shrunken market for your products and services.

An interruption in your business operations may mean that vendors are unable to make deliveries, employees can't report to work, or customers are unable to reach you. It may put you in violation of regulatory or contractual obligations, resulting in fines and penalties. It may cause you to lose market share.

Have a contingency plan for your business that will help you to restore infrastructure components when they are significantly impacted by a disaster and will give you the ability to keep essential business operations running. Depending on the type of business you operate, you may need a manufacturing facility for receiving, production, and shipping. You will also need the capability to communicate with vendors and customers, via phone, email, and your website. You will need to protect your cash flow, including a means to issue payroll to employees and to track transactions with vendors and customers.

Assess the risks for your business, taking into account the natural and man-made disasters to which your business is most vulnerable. Are you susceptible to hurricanes? Flooding? Tornadoes? Wildfires? Earthquakes? Are you close to a nuclear power facility or a plant that produces hazardous chemicals? Mitigate for the most likely disaster first, and then prepare for others.

❑ Develop an emergency plan with the following goals:

- Protect employees, visitors, and assets of the business such as equipment and inventory, computer system, and paper files.

- Have a means to temporarily replace tools, equipment, supplies, and outside services you would need to keep operations running.

❑ Establish timelines and budgets for accomplishing the goals of your emergency plan.

❑ Form an emergency-management team. Assign specifics tasks to each member of the team, such as maintaining first aid supplies, marking evacuation routes, maintaining fire extinguishers, etc.

❑ Create an emergency-control center with the following:

- Copy of emergency management plan, including names and phone numbers of all members of the emergency management team
- Contact information for police, fire department, hospitals, local/state/federal emergency management agencies, hazardous materials response team, national weather service, utility companies (water, gas, electric)
- Facility map, including drawings of utilities and security system, evacuation routes, hazardous materials, etc.
- Generator for backup power
- Communications equipment, including a NOAA radio
- Sanitation station
- First aid station
- Food and water

❑ Establish staging areas inside your facility, as well as outside, in case evacuation of the building is necessary. Designated members of your management team should be assigned to take a head count for each department, so that all employees can be accounted for in case the building must be evacuated.

❑ Put your plan in writing and distribute it to all employees so they know what to do in case of an emergency. Conduct orientation and educational sessions for employees to familiarize them with your emergency procedures.

❑ Provide training, not only in the proper use of your equipment, but also in first aid and CPR.

❑ Maintain your equipment and your surroundings to create a safe working environment.

❑ Practice your emergency responsiveness with drills.

❑ Establish policies that minimize the opportunities for workplace violence:

  ◆ Keep company vehicles locked. Encourage employees to keep their private vehicles locked.

  ◆ Keep all gates and outside entry doors locked during the day, if possible.

  ◆ Require visitors to check in and be escorted at all times while on the premises.

❑ Back up your computer files on a regular basis. How many transactions or hours of work can you afford to lose? That's how often you should back up. Then store the backups offsite. You can subscribe to an online data storage service, but in case of a widespread problem with the power grid or the Internet, your data might be unavailable to you. Make your own backups and store them offsite where they will be readily available to you.

❑ Make sure your insurance includes "business income coverage" and "extra expense insurance" so your livelihood won't be destroyed by a disaster. If your building is damaged, would you be able to make the mortgage payment as well as a rent payment on temporary quarters? Would you be able to pay utilities at both locations? Would you have enough money to replace damaged inventory, equipment, and office furnishings? Other considerations may include moving expenses, ongoing expenses of the business such as advertising that was already contracted before the disaster occurred, and lost profits.

FINANCIAL COLLAPSE

Financial disaster can result from a loss of assets, a loss of income, or incurring a large liability such as medical expenses. If you rely on a job for your income, a fire that burns down your place of employment could be a financial disaster. If you rely on mutual funds for your income, a crash in the stock market could be a financial disaster. If you rely on rental property for your income, a flood could be a financial disaster. You could become disabled and unable to work, lose your spouse, or suffer other devastating events that cause a major interruption in your income.

- Keep your finances in order. Make survival planning a part of your household budgeting and financial planning. Live within your means, stay out of debt, and set aside savings for emergencies.

- Keep your job skills current. Take continuing education courses so you will always have the skills employers are looking for in your field.

- Maintain a network of professional contacts who can help you find a job if you lose your current one. If the company you work for is financially unstable, don't wait to be laid off with everyone else; get out and find a new job before everyone else starts looking.

- Keep enough money stashed away to cover at least six months of living expenses, enough to pay your mortgage or rent, utilities, vehicle payments, insurance, and groceries. If you lose your job through no fault of your own, you would be covered by unemployment insurance, but it pays only a fraction of your regular wage.

- If case of long-term unemployment, have a contingency plan. Be prepared to share living expenses with a friend or relative. Use your skills for part-time or temporary work. Develop a skill set that is unrelated to your current profession so you can go in a different direction if you need to.

- Buy adequate property insurance to cover your home, vehicles, and personal property.

- Buy health insurance to cover major medical expenses.

- Set aside cash to cover the insurance deductibles. If you file a claim, that money will still be coming out of your pocket, but you won't notice it as much if it doesn't disrupt your regular budget.

- Buy disability insurance to cover your lost income if you become disabled and can't work.

- Buy life insurance to provide for your spouse and children if you die.

- Beware of scams. Have a secret password that no one would be able to guess, and share this password with the members of your group. Require this password from any stranger who contacts you with a request for money to help your loved ones, claiming they need money for bail, legal fees, medical treatment, car repairs, etc.

- Diversify your investments so that if one sector crashes, you won't be totally wiped out.

BASIC SKILLS

In an emergency, you may have to rely on yourself for survival. Others, especially your children, may also rely on you for their survival. The more knowledge and experience you have, the greater your chances for success. The world is full of opportunities to expand your skills. Become a life-long learner.

- ◆ Participate in sports that teach you practical skills that you could use in an emergency situation. Learn how to swim, how to paddle a canoe, how to hoist a sail, and how to snow ski.

- ◆ Grow a garden.

- ◆ Study martial arts and learn self-defense.

- ◆ Learn how to drive a vehicle with a manual transmission.

- ◆ Take a sewing class. Learn how to sew a seam and make your own garments.

- ◆ Learn first aid and CPR.

- ◆ Take a cooking class.

- ◆ Learn how to make pottery.

- ◆ Volunteer with a service organization and learn basic carpentry, plumbing, and electrical skills.

Personal Practices

❑ Get in shape with proper nutrition, exercise, and sleep.

❑ Get vaccinated and keep your vaccinations up to date.

❑ Observe good personal hygiene habits.

❑ Observe safe food-handling practices.

❑ Observe safe mail-handling practices.

❑ Be careful when you travel.

- ◆ Let someone know where you are going.
- ◆ Stay on main roads, and stay in a trusted hotel.
- ◆ Travel with others and be observant of your surroundings.

❑ Maintain your vehicle and keep the fuel tank full.

❑ Stay informed about weather conditions.

❑ If you own a business, develop an emergency plan for it.
  ❑ Form an emergency-management team.
  ❑ Create an emergency-control center.
  ❑ Establish staging areas to account for employees.
  ❑ Provide training to your employees.
  ❑ Back up your computer files.
  ❑ Review your insurance coverage.

❑ Keep your personal finances in order.

❑ Keep your job skills current, and develop alternate skill sets.

❑ Buy insurance.

❑ Learn practical life skills by participating in sports, taking classes, and pursuing hobbies to broaden your knowledge.

Chapter 7

Recovery Plan

This chapter outlines what you can do before a disaster strikes to help you with the recovery process afterward. It primarily involves maintaining documentation of who you are and what you have so your life can be restored to "normal" as quickly as possible after a disaster.

❑ Carry identification with you. After a widespread disaster, you may have to prove where you live before you will be allowed to return to your neighborhood.

❑ Use a scrolling tool to inscribe the last four digits of your social security number on expensive items to aid in their identification if stolen.

❑ Create a written inventory of all of your possessions, and take photos of your home and possessions for insurance purposes in case you need to make a claim. Keep a set of hardcopy printouts and electronic files with you at home, and store another set offsite.

❑ Save receipts for major purchases such as furniture, appliances, electronics, antiques, artwork, jewelry, and furs. Also save receipts for less expensive items that are part of a collection and that together represent a substantial sum of money.

❑ For all of your important papers, scan copies onto your computer. Keep one hardcopy set of documents at home and a second set at another location.

Electronic files are crucial if your old-fashioned paper documents are lost or destroyed during a disaster. On the other hand, those old-fashioned paper documents are critical if your computer files are destroyed or you don't have access to a working computer during or after a crisis.

❑ Make regular backups of computer files on flash drives and store one copy where it can be readily accessed and store another copy offsite, preferably out of your area. Set up an exchange system with a long-distance friend or relative: you keep their data, they keep yours.

Build redundancy into your system by subscribing to an online service for data storage that you can access from any computer.

❑ Practice computer safety.

◆ Restrict access to your computer.

◆ Use passwords on all computer files.

◆ Install a firewall.

◆ Install antivirus software.

◆ Do not download files from any site or open any email attachment unless you are absolutely sure the source is trustworthy.

◆ Do not provide any personal information such as social security number, bank account number, or passwords to anyone you don't know personally or regularly do business with.

❑ Keep important papers and computer backup media in a water-resistant, fire-resistant, impact-resistant safe. Sure, copies of your documents are available at the court house, bureau of motor vehicles, bank, etc., but only if those places are functioning entities; if they're closed because of a disaster, you'll be on your own to provide any documentation you need.

Safes come in various classes, such as 125, 150, and 350; the number refers to degrees Fahrenheit. They are rated against fire for 30 minutes up to four hours. (After the specified amount of time, heat transfer will turn papers to ash.) So a Class 125 safe rated for four hours will keep your materials at a lower temperature for a longer time than a Class 350 safe rated for one hour. If you don't have a safe, put your documents in plastic and store them in the freezer; this doesn't provide as much protection as a safe, but it may provide a little.

❑   Review your insurance coverage.

Homeowner's Insurance

Basic policies cover perils such as windstorm and hail, fire and lightning, smoke, explosion, volcanic eruption, glass breakage, damage from vehicles, vandalism, civil disturbances, and theft. Riders provide additional coverage (and additional premiums!) for earthquakes, hurricanes, terrorism, war, and other hazards. Flood insurance is not included in a typical homeowner's policy. The federal government provides flood insurance through private companies that sell and service flood insurance policies. Ask your insurance agent or insurance company for more information.

Make sure you understand what kinds of hazards are covered. Some policies list only events that are included. Other policies list only events that are excluded.

Also make sure you understand what benefits you will receive from the policy.

Home value: Some policies are written to cover only the purchase price that you paid for your house, while others are written to cover replacement value. Verify that you are carrying enough insurance to cover the loss of your home.

Loss of use covers the additional expenses of living in a hotel or rental property while your home is being repaired.

Liability insurance covers your financial responsibilities to others for bodily injury caused while they are on your property, and property damage caused to others by members of your household.

You may be able to lower your premiums if you can demonstrate to the insurer that you have taken measures to mitigate damage to your property.

Landlord insurance

This insurance provides essentially the same benefits as homeowner's insurance, but it applies to property that is rented to others.

Personal Property Insurance

Many homeowner policies cover the "contents" of your home, including furniture, appliances, clothing, electronics, jewelry, furs, tools, etc. This is the same coverage provided by a tenants' policy for someone who rents.

Such a policy typically provides a flat amount of coverage for each category of personal possessions, even if you have receipts to prove that you spent more than the scheduled values. For instance, if your house burns down, you may lose $20,000 worth of flat-screen TVs, audio equipment, computers, and gaming systems, but if your policy provides only $10,000 worth of coverage for electronics, $10k is all you're going to get no matter how many receipts you produce. Your insurance company will be happy to sell you additional coverage above and beyond what's included in the base policy, but it's relatively expensive. You'll have to decide whether it's worth it to you to pay the extra premium, or assume more of the risk yourself.

Also, be aware that if you make a claim, your property will be depreciated before the insurance company makes a payout. You may have $10,000 worth of coverage for electronics and $10k in receipts, but your insurance company may pay only $8,000 of your claim because your stuff is *old* and *used*.

Vehicle Insurance (cars, boats, recreational vehicles, etc.)

The three basic components of vehicle insurance are:

Liability insurance: covers your financial responsibilities to others for bodily injury and property damage caused by the vehicle.

Medical insurance: covers costs for treating your own injuries and undergoing rehabilitation. This may duplicate other health insurance you have.

Property insurance: covers damage or loss of your own vehicle from fire, theft, or collision.

Other optional coverage includes emergency road service, car rental and travel expense, death, dismemberment, and loss of sight, disability, uninsured motorist, use of non-owned vehicles, and loss of earnings.

Health Insurance

Health insurance policies may be provided by your employer, or you may purchase them on your own. They provide a wide range of benefits, and therefore come with a wide range of premiums. The three basic components of health insurance are:

- major medical

- dental

- vision

Disability Insurance

Workers' compensation insurance, paid for by your employer, covers your medical expenses and part of your wages for an illness or injury incurred while at work.

Private disability insurance provides financial support if you are unable to work due to an illness or injury that is not work-related. These policies may be provided by your employer, or you may purchase them on your own.

Short-term disability insurance generally provides benefits for three to six months.

Long-term disability benefits usually start when short-term disability benefits end, and generally last up to 12 months.

After 12 months, if you are considered permanently disabled, social security benefits may be available to you. In this case, you would contact the federal Social Security Administration.

Life Insurance

If you have a spouse, children, or others who are dependent on you financially, you should have life insurance. When you die, the proceeds of the policy can be paid in a lump sum or in annuity payments.

Crop insurance

This insurance protects farmers against weather damage, insects, and disease.

Livestock insurance

This insurance typically protects owners against loss from accident, illness, or disease.

Pet insurance

This insurance is generally health insurance for accidents and illnesses, but can also include burial.

Other insurance

Virtually any kind of risk can be insured. If you have questions, ask the person who is providing the product or service you wish to insure. This is just a partial list of other coverage that may be available:

- directors & officers liability insurance
- errors & omissions insurance
- professional liability insurance
- pollution insurance
- mortgage insurance
- credit insurance
- title insurance
- travel insurance
- expatriate insurance
- kidnap & ransom insurance
- legal expense insurance
- extended warranties

❑ Have enough cash or savings to pay all of your deductibles:

- Real estate insurance deductibles $_____
- Personal property insurance deductibles $_____
- Vehicle insurance deductibles $_____
- Health insurance deductibles $_____
- Other insurance deductibles $_____

Recovery Plan

❏ Carry identification with you so authorities will allow you back home.

❏ Use a scrolling tool to inscribe the last four digits of your social security number on expensive items.

❏ Inventory your possessions; keep a set of hardcopy printouts and electronic files with you at home, and store another set offsite.

❏ Save receipts.

❏ Scan important documents onto your computer. Keep one hardcopy set of documents at home and a second set at another location.

❏ Make regular backups of computer files on flash drives and store one copy where it can be readily accessed and store another copy offsite, preferably out of your area.

❏ Practice computer safety.

♦ Restrict access to your computer.

♦ Use passwords on all computer files.

♦ Install a firewall.

♦ Install antivirus software.

♦ Do not download files from any site or open any email attachment unless you are absolutely sure the source is trustworthy.

♦ Do not provide any personal information to anyone you don't know.

❏ Keep important papers and computer backup media in a water-resistant, fire-resistant, impact-resistant safe.

❏ Review your insurance coverage.

❏ Have enough cash or savings to pay all of your deductibles.

Documents & Valuables to store (hardcopies & electronic media)

_____ birth certificates
_____ death certificates
_____ marriage certificates
_____ divorce decrees
_____ adoption papers
_____ custody or guardianship papers
_____ selective service registrations
_____ military discharge papers
_____ passports, visas, naturalization records
_____ social security account numbers
_____ voter registrations
_____ college transcripts, diplomas, certifications, licenses
_____ property deeds
_____ vehicle titles and vehicle registrations
_____ drivers' licenses or other state-issued identification
_____ proof of residence (utility bill, property tax record)
_____ checking account numbers with institution names & phone numbers
_____ savings account numbers with institution names & phone numbers
_____ retirement account numbers with institution names & phone numbers
_____ brokerage account numbers with institution names & phone numbers
_____ credit card account numbers with institution names & phone numbers
_____ stock certificates
_____ bond certificates
_____ contracts
_____ wills, trusts, powers of attorney, medical directives
_____ mortgages, vehicle loans, personal loans
_____ insurance policies (health, disability, life, real estate, vehicles)
_____ prepaid funeral contract and burial plot deed
_____ tax records (3 years)
_____ vaccination records
_____ medical histories, allergies, chronic conditions
_____ prescriptions for eyeglasses and medications
_____ household inventory, with photos
_____ receipts for major purchases, major home improvement records
_____ warranties
_____ jewelry
_____ precious metals
_____ spare keys for home and vehicles

Chapter 8

Apocalypse Plan

No one likes to think about what could happen to their lives and their loved ones in a major catastrophe, but the chances that you will be affected by such a calamity are increasing. Hurricanes and tornadoes are becoming stronger and more frequent. Viruses and bacteria are becoming more virulent. Earthquakes are happening in parts of the country that haven't seen seismic activity in centuries. The headlines every day are about workplace violence, chemical spills, and infrastructure breakdowns. Droughts occur in one part of the country and floods in another, destroying food and ruining livelihoods.

Nuclear winter (caused by the detonation of nuclear weapons), impact winter (caused by a comet or asteroid hitting the earth), and volcanic winter (caused by a supervolcano eruption) describe climate changes that might occur in catastrophic circumstances. If the atmosphere were filled with dust clouds and/or smoke, blocking the sun's light for months or even years, temperatures would drop, precipitation would decrease, crops would fail, and livestock would perish, causing widespread starvation.

Imagine if a catastrophe wiped out a significant portion of our population. It wouldn't just mean fewer people. What if there weren't enough qualified people to maintain all of our nuclear power facilities, for instance? You can't just flip a switch and turn those babies off. Who would maintain dams, power generating stations, and transmission lines? Who would maintain oil refineries and gas and oil pipelines? Who would maintain sewage treatment facilities? Who would maintain ships and seaports, planes and airports? Who would maintain the trucks that bring us goods, the highways they travel on, and the bridges they cross?

We rely on energy in various forms to heat and cool our homes, pump our water and sewage, cook our food, provide our transportation, and keep us connected to the world through TV, the Internet, and our cell phones. Without widespread power over a prolonged period of time, we would go back to living like it's the 1800's, before the Industrial Revolution.

In the face of these possibilities, the best thing to do is to prepare for the worst-case scenario. The worst thing that can happen isn't necessarily the most likely thing that will happen, but if you're prepared for the worst, then you can deal with anything less than that.

Get back to the basics and develop core survival skills. Know how to produce your own food and construct your own shelter. Ideally, every teen and adult member of your group should know all of the skills needed to survive. Even young children can learn simple skills.

One approach to acquiring these skills is to learn each one together as a group. The disadvantage to this approach is that in the beginning your group is not diversified in its skill set. On the upside, training together can be a good bonding experience. Skills such as using a compass or applying basic first aid lend themselves well to group training.

Another approach is to assign each group member a set of skills to learn and then teach to the other members of the group. This is also a good bonding experience, as one person becomes the specialist and teaches the others the basics. Skills that require specialization, such as operating computer hardware and software, lend themselves well to this approach.

If complete cross-training isn't feasible, divide the skills among the group members so that as a whole, you'll have all of the skills you need to survive.

Start by reading background information, and then get hands-on experience with the skill. You can do this on your own, by taking individual or group instruction for a single skill, or by attending a survival camp that teaches multiple skills. Tent camping at a primitive site (no RV's, no electricity, and no running water!) can provide an opportunity to catch a fish, scale it, build a fire, and cook the fish for a meal. If you've never fired a weapon, have a qualified marksman show you the proper way to handle a firearm, and then put in some time on your own at a firing range to improve your aim.

The topics in this chapter are:
- personnel
- animals
- navigation skills
- firemaking
- shelter
- water purification
- food
- clothing
- security
- money
- marketable skills
- library

PERSONNEL

In the case of a life-altering catastrophic event where survival becomes a long-term endeavor, it may be beneficial to be part of a larger group where several strong adults can share the heaviest parts of the workload. However, making your immediate family part of a larger group will be beneficial only if the group can function well together. This may be possible with extended family members such as grandparents, adult siblings, and cousins, or even close friends. But if your relatives are jerks (you know which ones I'm talking about), you're better off not forming an alliance with them. Everyone has to be willing to contribute and to cooperate.

Once you have decided whom to include in your group, assign duties to each group member. The person designated becomes *primarily* responsible for the duty specified, but is not *solely* responsible. The other group members must be willing to share all aspects of the workload, and not work just in their own areas of responsibility. In the list below, the dietician, for instance, is responsible for the group's food supply. That does not mean this person has exclusive responsibility for acquiring and preparing food. Other group members must help draw water, harvest crops, cook meals, clean the kitchen, and do whatever else is required to feed the group. The dietician, as the "head cheese" in the area of food, coordinates these activities and makes sure the group is always fed.

Every member of your group should be able to perform most of these duties at a basic level. For example, everyone should know how to operate the two-way radio, even though only one person will have primary responsibility for operating, maintaining, and repairing it. In the beginning, it's unlikely that every member of your group will be able to perform every duty. To get you started, divide the skills among the members of your group so that as a whole, you will learn all of the skills you need to survive in as short a period as possible. Then over time, everyone can cross-train on the other skills they need to develop.

Learning new skills and upgrading existing skills is an ongoing process. Set weekly goals for each group member to learn a new skill or upgrade on existing one. Schedule hands-on training for skills such as using a compass, a chainsaw, or a rifle. Schedule problem-solving exercises such as foraging for food, tracking animals, or building a shelter. The more you train, the more confident you will become, and survival is all about confidence.

After training, reward your group by having dinner together or enjoying some other leisure-time activity together. Not only does it give group members an incentive to work hard, but it also helps bond the group members to one another. Cohesiveness is another important ingredient in survival.

To minimize conflict and finger-pointing, avoid overlapping responsibilities. The dietician and medic are both responsible for the health of the group members, but in different ways. They must each have clearly defined areas of responsibility. For instance, water is consumed internally and used for washing. You could make the dietician responsible for the drinking water and make the medic responsible for the water used for washing, but if you have only one water source, it makes more sense to put one person in charge of the sanitation of the entire water system.

All members of the group need to feel they have a valuable contribution to make. All members of the group, including young children, the elderly, and the disabled, should be assigned some task to perform, no matter how small.

Following are some examples of roles that need to be filled. You can rearrange the responsibilities of these positions to suit the members of your group. It doesn't matter who does what, as long as the areas of responsibility are clearly defined and all necessary tasks are accomplished. For small groups, group members will have to assume more than one role.

Group Leader – coordinates group activities; evaluates data and directs appropriate responses; arbitrates disputes between group members; serves as spokesperson when dealing with others outside the group

Engineer – oversees demolition or construction of any structure needed, such as shelters for people and animals, cellars or bins for food storage, cisterns, wells, fences, roads, bridges, and transport vehicles; knows how to run plumbing and wiring and how to design, operate, and repair machinery

Power Specialist – generates power by whatever means are available (water, wind, solar, gasoline, diesel, coal, wood, biofuels, dung); maintains and repairs generator, batteries, and other power-related equipment

Information & Communications Specialist – responsible for operation and maintenance of computers, radio receivers and transmitters, and other devices; conducts research; communicates with outside groups; maintains library of reference books

Dietician – responsible for the food supply; cultivates plants, harvests wild plants; preserves fruits and vegetables; coordinates trapping, hunting, and fishing; coordinates feeding livestock, milking cows, gathering eggs, etc.

Medic – administers first aid; sets broken limbs and performs minor surgery; knows how to collect and purify water; responsible for sanitation, including monitoring the purity of the water supply, maintenance of latrines, and manure control; leads group exercises to maintain physical fitness

Weapons Specialist – procures and issues weapons; maintains the group's arsenal, cleaning and repairing weapons; reloads ammunition; maintains storehouse of explosives

Security Specialist – secures and monitors perimeter of compound; trains and cares for guard dogs and attack dogs; analyzes intelligence

Firefighters – oversee proper storage of hazardous materials; suppress fires with fire extinguishers, dirt, or water

Logistician – procures supplies and arranges transport; tracks inventory of materials, tools, vehicles, etc.; maintains and repairs tools and vehicles

Financial Specialist – coordinates projects to generate income for group; collects and disburses funds as needed to fulfill duties of all group members

ANIMALS

Be prepared to make use of animals.

Dogs. Dogs can herd other animals, pull or carry loads, rescue people in distress, lead the blind and aid the disabled, hunt, patrol, attack, and sniff out explosives or drugs.

Cats. Cats can help control pests such as mice.

Horses, mules, donkeys, oxen. Beasts of burden can carry you or other loads or can pull wagons, carts, and plows. Tie a bell or tin cans to a horse's halter and the movement of his head will warn you if danger approaches. Manure can be used for fertilizer or dried for fuel.

Cows, goats, sheep. These animals can provide milk, meat, wool, and leather as well as fertilizer.

Pigs. Pigs provide both meat and leather.

Rabbits. Rabbits provide meat and fur. (And good luck charms!)

Birds. Chickens, ducks, and geese provide eggs, meat, and feathers. Geese also make good alarm animals. Pigeons can carry messages.

Bees. Bees pollinate crops and provide honey.

Earthworms. Worms aerate the soil and make good fish bait.

NAVIGATION SKILLS

In an apocalyptic situation, you may be able to stay in your present home and geographic area, but it is also possible that you will have to relocate, either because your home is uninhabitable, or you need to search for resources outside of your immediate area.

If you have a GPS and the satellites are still working, you will have a good navigational aid as long as you have power for the device. You can follow existing roads, but only as long as they are safe for passage.

❑ Learn to navigate with a compass, the sun, and the stars. Take a class or buy a book on the subject, and go out in the wilderness to practice your skills.

FIREMAKING

In a survival situation, hypothermia is one of the greatest threats to your life, so knowing how to make fire is a critical skill. A fire is versatile: it provides not only warmth, but also light, a way to cook food, and protection from predators. In addition, the crackling sound and aroma of burning wood provide comfort. Common ways to start a fire are with:

- **friction** using a hand drill, bow drill, pump drill, or similar device; this is a difficult technique and takes practice, but once you know how to do it, you'll always be able to make fire

- **flint-and-steel**, **ferrocerium,** or **magnesium fire starter**

- **steel wool** and a **battery**

- **matches**

- **butane lighter**

- **clear lens** or **mirror** that is used to focus energy from the sun on the tinder

Using combinations of certain chemicals to start a fire is possible but too dangerous for amateurs, and may be illegal in some circumstances, so you won't see a list of those compounds in this manual.

For a wood fire, you'll need three grades of material:

- **tinder** – the smallest pieces, used to start the fire, such as crushed leaves, thin pieces of bark, or dried grass

- **kindling** – the middle–sized pieces, used to build up the fire, such as small twigs and branches

- **fuel** – the largest pieces, used to keep the fire burning, such as split logs

To build a fire, start with the tinder, add kindling, and then add fuel. Give each stage time to burn and become hot enough to ignite the next largest pieces of wood.

❑ Practice starting a fire using various methods.

SHELTER

Along with being able to build a fire, being able to build a shelter is a vital survival skill. A shelter will help you survive the elements of heat, cold, wind, and precipitation. The kind of shelter you build depends on what materials are available, how quickly you need to have it, and how long you will be using it. If the sun is going down or a storm is approaching, you'll be limited in how much time you can spend on it. If you're on the move and will be using the shelter for only one night, you'll want to limit the amount of energy you expend on constructing it.

A temporary shelter may be a natural formation that you seek out, such as a snow bank, a rock overhang, a downed tree, a hollow stump, or a cave.

A temporary shelter can also be a tent or tarp that you carry with you, or something that you make out of available materials, taking shape as a lean-to, a wickiup or wigwam, a tipi, a tree-house, or an igloo.

A permanent shelter may take shape as an adobe hut, a log cabin, a stone house, an underground or partially earth-sheltered dwelling, or many other forms, depending on the materials you have available and the skills you have.

❑ Practice by going out into the wilderness and looking for natural formations that you could use as a temporary shelter in an emergency. Be sure to look for wildlife (snakes! scorpions! coyotes! bears!) before forging ahead.

❑ Practice erecting a tent.

❑ Practice building a temporary shelter from tree branches, rocks, or whatever is available to you. (If you do this on private land, be sure you have the owner's permission. If you do this on public land, be sure you restore the habitat to its natural state; "take only pictures, leave only footprints.")

❑ To develop the skills for building a permanent shelter, practice using hand tools and power tools. Take on some do-it-yourself projects around the house, such as setting tile, installing an electrical fixture, and performing simple plumbing repairs. Participate in hobbies such as woodworking and metalworking.

WATER PURIFICATION

Temporary water-treatment methods generally produce only a small amount of potable water and are not suitable for long-term needs. In an apocalyptic situation, once you have settled down, you will need a permanent water-purification system.

Water purification relies on gravity or a pump to run water through a series of filters that remove progressively smaller particles. As the final step, the water is chemically treated to kill any remaining bacteria or viruses.

A basic water purification system may include the following:

- screen on the intake pipe at the water source to filter out large debris

- settling tank where large particles settle out of the water

- series of filters where smaller particles are trapped

    - top layer: big rocks
    - 4th layer: little rocks
    - 3rd layer: coarse gravel
    - 2nd layer: fine gravel
    - bottom layer: sand

- holding tank where chlorine is added to kill bacteria and viruses

To get an idea of how such a system works, tour a water treatment facility.

FOOD

Famine may result from a drought, a flood, freezing temperatures, pestilence, or a nuclear holocaust. Or food may be available, but too expensive to buy because of a widespread economic catastrophe.

❑ Store food today for long-term future use. If stored properly, staples can last for several years. Ideally, you should have two years' worth of nonperishable food for each member of your group. This will give you enough time to relocate, if necessary, and start growing your own food. If this sounds extreme, consider this: If an earth-changing catastrophe happened in the summer and you were forced to move, you may not be able to plant crops until the following spring. Then it would be several more months before you would see any yield. You could easily be consuming the second year of your stockpile before your crops yield enough food to sustain you and your family.

However, storing food is only a temporary solution. Eventually, your stock would run out, and you would have to find ways to replenish your food supply. This means either forage for edible plants, grow and harvest your own crops, kill game, or raise your own livestock.

❑ Take trips out into the wilderness with a field guide for edible plants and learn to identify what you can eat. When you travel, make it a point to learn about what's available in other geographic areas.

❑ Grow your own food in the current season, and stockpile seeds for the next growing season. Even if you don't need to rely on raising your own crops for your food supply now, it's a good idea to practice your horticultural skills so you'll know how to successfully raise crops if the need arises. You don't need acreage to do this; if you live in a small space, practice container gardening.

If you plant your own garden to raise your own fruits and vegetables, be sure to use non-hybrid seeds, which regenerate. Hybrid seeds grow plants only once; the seeds from these plants are sterile and will not produce food the following season.

❑ Trap, hunt, or fish for food. As with growing crops, even if you don't need to rely on trapping, hunting, and fishing for your food supply now, it's a good idea to practice those skills so you'll be able to put food on the table with those methods if the need arises.

❑ Start raising your own livestock. Virtually anyone can raise fish, since they don't make noise and won't bother your neighbors. Some communities allow fowl (chickens, ducks, geese, and turkeys), rabbits, and bees to be housed within the city limits. If size is an issue, you may be able to keep smaller breeds, such as pygmy goats or miniature cattle. Some local laws allow "pets" but not "livestock," so if you name your goat and call it a "pet," you'll be allowed to keep it (and milk it!); check with your local authorities regarding restrictions. (Restrictions are usually related to noise, smell, and sanitation. If you can address those issues, you'll be allowed to keep your animals.) If you live outside the city limits, you can raise larger breeds as well as a larger variety of animals.

❑ In addition to producing food, you'll need to preserve what you don't eat right away. Refer to a cookbook or a survivalist's manual to develop skills for preserving food such as canning, drying, and pickling.

If you plan to raise crops or livestock in an apocalyptic environment, be prepared to guard and protect your resources 24/7.

CLOTHING

One of the things we take most for granted in modern society is our clothing. We can cook without our microwaves, and we can communicate without our cell phones and computers, but what would we do without our clothes? Sure, we could make our own clothes; many people today do. *But what about the cloth?*

If an apocalyptic event knocked us back to a time before our 20th- and 21st- century technologies, we wouldn't have the luxury of powered looms to create cloth for us. We would be back to spinning thread and weaving cloth by hand, both time-consuming and labor-intensive endeavors.

Clothing can be made from a variety of materials: leather, fur, wool, silk, cotton, flax, and other plant fibers.

❏ Learn how to skin animals and prepare the hides. If this sounds like more than you want to take on personally (!), visit a tannery or at the very least, get a book on the subject so you could do it if you *had* to.

❏ Take up spinning and weaving as hobbies, or visit spinning and weaving hobbyists for a demonstration to see how it's done.

❏ Take up knitting and crocheting as hobbies. Make gifts for your family and friends to practice your skills.

SECURITY

Stockpile weapons and ammunition to be used for hunting food and self-defense. You must be prepared to defend your own life and the lives of your loved ones, and to defend the resources that support your lives. Such resources could include livestock, crops, medicine, or wood to burn for warmth.

Build your arsenal with a variety of weapons, but only those you are willing and able to use. Weapons can be lethal or non-lethal. They include a wide range of tools, such as pepper spray, stun guns, batons, slingshots, spears, harpoons, knives, swords, bows, firearms, and explosives.

Your choice of weapons depends on your abilities, your strengths and weaknesses, and your anticipated needs. Check the laws in your state regarding restrictions for any weapon that you want to carry.

Get training from professionals so you'll know how to correctly use your weapons of choice. Practice using them. Weapons are worthless, or dangerous to you, if you don't know how to use them properly.

Stock up on ammunition. Ammunition may become scarce, and what good is a gun if you don't have any bullets? Learn to load your own ammunition and buy the supplies to do so.

Having a wide variety of firearms at your disposal may seem like a good idea, but it complicates your life. Limiting your arsenal to a few standard types of firearms serves two purposes: one, you reduce the variety of ammunition you have to keep on hand, and two, if one weapon breaks, you can use it for spare parts for another one.

For firearms, as a minimum, have a handgun, a rifle, and a shotgun.

Pro's and con's of shotguns:
♦ effective against close, moving targets
♦ effective against small targets
♦ relatively easy to hit your target
♦ versatile ammunition (a single slug or a wide range of pellet sizes)
♦ ineffective at long distances
♦ heavy to carry

Pro's and con's of rifles:
- effective against long-range targets
- less recoil than a shotgun
- require precise aim to be effective

Pro's and con's of revolvers:
- can handle a wide variety of ammunition
- can handle larger cartridges that have greater stopping power
- readiness to fire due to lack of safety device
- less likely to jam due to mechanical simplicity
- spent cartridges remain in the cylinder for easy retrieval
- easy to maintain
- lack of safety device can lead to accidental discharges
- subject to hang fire
- require precise aim to be effective
- carries less ammunition than a pistol

Pro's and con's of pistols:
- larger ammunition capacity of magazine (vs. a revolver cylinder)
- faster to reload
- less expensive ammunition (usually)
- lighter trigger pull than a revolver
- less recoil than a revolver
- compact design and lighter weight make them easier to carry
- safety device can help prevent accidental discharges
- slight delay in readiness to fire due to safety device
- require precise aim to be effective
- if it jams, shooter must know how to clear it

Pro's and con's of hand bows:
- quieter than firearms
- faster reloading than a crossbow
- lighter than a crossbow

Pro's and con's of crossbows:
- quieter than firearms
- more powerful than a hand bow
- smaller than a hand bow
- heavier than a hand bow
- slower reloading than a hand bow

MONEY

Our money works as an exchange medium because people have faith in our financial system. But if that system breaks down for any reason, our paper currency will become virtually worthless. This could happen as the result of a widespread event or series of events, such as a pandemic, drought or flooding that wipes out crops, or damage to significant parts of our infrastructure. Anything that causes widespread civil unrest and a breakdown in our institutions and government authority will lead to a collapse of the financial system as well.

If this happens, our exchange media may become commodities such as gold or silver, because they have intrinsic value. So besides stockpiling currency, either in the form of cash or a bank account, it may be wise to put some of your assets into precious metals.

But if people become truly desperate, even gold and silver will become worthless. In a survival situation, people will be looking for things that will sustain their lives, and these are the items that will be most valuable:

♦ water and water-purification supplies and equipment
♦ food, especially staples such as flour, rice, beans, cooking oil, canned goods, coffee, tea
♦ seeds and garden tools
♦ canning supplies, such as jars, lids, sealing rings
♦ chickens, cows, goats, sheep, dogs
♦ fishing rods and lures, nets, spears
♦ cookware, especially cast iron
♦ insulated coolers/ice chests
♦ medical supplies
♦ eyeglasses
♦ personal hygiene supplies such as toothbrushes and toothpaste, soap, feminine hygiene products
♦ sanitation supplies such as toilet paper, garbage bags, cleaners, laundry detergent, bleach
♦ pest control, such as insect repellent, poison, traps
♦ building materials for shelter against the elements, such as tarps, rope, stakes, lumber, stone
♦ fuel, such as wood, gasoline, propane cylinders
♦ clothing to stay warm, work clothes such as heavy boots and gloves, raingear

- fabric and sewing supplies
- blankets, pillows, sleeping bags, cots, mattresses
- backpacks, duffel bags
- lighting devices with wicks/matches/fuel, batteries, etc.
- manual utensils, tools, and equipment
- hardware such as nails, nuts and bolts, screws
- duct tape
- powered equipment, especially generators and chain saws
- anything solar-powered
- spare parts for machinery and equipment
- fire extinguishers or baking soda
- utility knives and sharpening stones
- weapons and ammunition, including firearms, bows, and knives
- bicycles and spare parts
- wagons, handcarts
- non-electronic games and toys
- alcohol, tobacco, gum, candy
- religious texts

People may resort to a pure barter system to get the things they need. (They may resort to thievery, too, which is why you need to be prepared to protect your resources 24/7.)

However, both parties have to want to trade at the same time and in the same place for bartering to work. If the guy down the road owns the only stand of trees around and you need firewood, you might offer him two chickens for a cord of wood. But if he doesn't want any chickens, or if he wants four chickens but you're only willing to give him two, it's no deal.

It doesn't matter whether you pay in cash or in chickens; the price of any product or service is what the buyer and seller agree on. Maybe instead of chickens, you have a spare pipe wrench that you're willing to trade and the other guy is willing to accept for a cord of wood. In a survivalist economy, anything and everything becomes "money."

If you aren't accustomed to bargaining for things, a good way to practice is to attend yard sales, flea markets, or auctions. Or join a barter co-op where you exchange your labor and expertise for goods and services that you need instead of paying cash for them. (Typical services include music lessons, tutoring, accounting services, legal services, babysitting, dog walking, and yard work.) Participating in activities like these will help you get a feel for what bartering is like and what goods and services are worth.

MARKETABLE SKILLS

As important as having tangible goods for trade is having a marketable skill. It goes with you wherever you go, so you can trade your labor and expertise for whatever you need, such as water, food, medicine, fuel, clothing, spare parts, etc.

Marketable skills that are likely to always be in demand include:

- medical
- engineering
- carpentry
- electrical
- mechanical
- plumbing
- welding
- metalworking
- electronics repair

Broaden your skill set by taking a class at a local community college, volunteering for a charitable organization, or tackling some do-it-yourself projects at home.

LIBRARY

Nobody knows how to do everything. Even if you have a well-rounded group, gaps in your knowledge are going to pop up here and there, so you'll need resources to fill in those gaps.

You can find out anything on the Internet (whether it's true or not!), but if your electricity is out, the Internet isn't going to do you any good as a resource. A portable computer can provide temporary access to the Internet, but that will last only as long as its battery is charged. Even if you have a generator, in the case of a widespread blackout, third-party servers may be down. So instead of relying on technology that may not be available in an emergency, build your own library of reference materials using good old-fashioned books.

Store your books where they will be readily accessible when you need them. For instance, store a first-aid manual with your medical supplies, and store an atlas in your vehicle.

Personnel

Group Leader _____

Engineer _____

Power Specialist _____

Information & Communication Specialist _____

Dietician _____

Medic _____

Weapons Specialist _____

Security Specialist _____

Firefighters _____

Logistician _____

Financial Specialist _____

_____ _____

_____ _____

_____ _____

_____ _____

_____ _____

_____ _____

_____ _____

_____ _____

Before Disaster

Skill	Name	Name	Name
Swim			
Build a fire			
Build a shelter			
Find & purify water			
Forage for food			
Raise crops			
Cook from scratch			
Catch & scale a fish			
Trap wild game			
Hunt wild game			
Dress wild game			
Preserve food by canning			
Administer first aid			
Administer CPR			
Celestial navigation			
Morse code			
Self-defense			
How to use firearms			
Reload ammunition			
How to use a bow			
Make clothing			

Skill	Name	Name	Name
Build a raft	_____	_____	_____
Sail	_____	_____	_____
Snow ski	_____	_____	_____
Basic carpentry	_____	_____	_____
Basic plumbing	_____	_____	_____
Basic wiring	_____	_____	_____
Basic welding	_____	_____	_____
How to tie knots	_____	_____	_____
_____	_____	_____	_____
_____	_____	_____	_____
_____	_____	_____	_____
_____	_____	_____	_____
_____	_____	_____	_____
_____	_____	_____	_____
_____	_____	_____	_____
_____	_____	_____	_____
_____	_____	_____	_____
_____	_____	_____	_____

Navigation

❑ Learn and practice navigation skills.

Firemaking

❑ Practice building a fire using primitive methods:

  ❑ friction using a hand drill, bow drill, pump drill, or similar device

  ❑ flint-and-steel, ferrocerium, or magnesium fire starter

  ❑ clear lens or mirror to focus energy from the sun on the tinder

Shelter

❑ Practice pitching a tent.

❑ Practice building various kinds of temporary shelters with materials in the environment:

  ❑ lean-to

  ❑ wickiup or wigwam

  ❑ tipi

  ❑ tree house

  ❑ igloo

❑ Develop basic carpentry, electrical, and plumbing skills.

Water

❑ Visit a water treatment facility to see how a basic filtering system works.

Food

❑ Store food for long-range needs.

❑ Learn how to forage for edible plants in the wild.

❑ Learn how to grow and harvest your own crops.

❑ Store seeds.

❑ Learn how to trap and hunt animals for food, as well as how to prepare them.

❑ Learn how to fish and how to prepare what you catch.

❑ Learn how to raise your own livestock.

❑ Learn how to preserve food by drying, canning, pickling, etc.

Clothing

- ❑ Visit a tannery and learn how to prepare hides.
- ❑ Visit spinning and weaving hobbyists for a demonstration on how to make yarn and cloth. Take up spinning and weaving as hobbies.
- ❑ Take up knitting and crocheting as hobbies.

Security

- ❑ Build your arsenal with a variety of weapons.
- ❑ Get training and practice.
- ❑ Stock up on ammunition.

Money

- ❑ Stockpile some precious metals, such as gold or silver.
- ❑ Attend yard sales, flea markets, or auctions to learn bartering.
- ❑ Join a barter co-op where you exchange your labor and expertise for goods and services that you need instead of paying cash for them.

Marketable Skills

- ❑ Broaden your skill set by taking a class at a local community college, volunteering for a charitable organization, or tackling some do-it-yourself projects at home.

Tools & Equipment

_____ compass
_____ GPS
_____ animal traps
_____ hunting knives
_____ fishing rods & reels, lures
_____ canning supplies
_____ spindle, spinning wheel
_____ loom
_____ knitting needles, crochet hooks

Security

_____ patrol dogs

_____ attack dogs

_____ binoculars

_____ pepper spray

_____ tear gas

_____ flash-bangs

_____ tactical balls

_____ stun gun

_____ baton

_____ spear

_____ harpoon

_____ sword

_____ bayonet

_____ combat knife

_____ bow & arrows

_____ slingshot

_____ sidearm & ammunition

_____ rifle with telescope & ammunition

_____ shotgun & ammunition

_____ reloading equipment & supplies

_____ explosives

_____ metal detector

_____ signal jammer

_____ night vision goggles

_____ handcuffs

_____ zip ties

_____ body armor

_____ rappelling harness

_____ camouflage body paint

Library

_____ first aid manual for humans

_____ first aid manual for animals

_____ maps or atlas

_____ bus routes, subway lines, rail networks, bike paths, hiking trails

_____ nautical charts

_____ Morse code

_____ international code of signals

_____ sign language

_____ astronomy and celestial navigation

_____ field guide to edible wild plants

_____ field guide to poisonous plants

_____ field guide to medicinal plants

_____ field guide to trees

_____ field guide to mammals

_____ field guide to birds

_____ field guide to insects

_____ field guide to amphibians and reptiles

_____ field guide to fish or marine life

_____ field guide to venomous animals

_____ field guide to rocks and minerals

_____ wilderness survival guide (building a shelter, building a fire, finding and purifying water, foraging for food, trapping and hunting food, etc.)

_____ basic construction and general repairs (plumbing, wiring, carpentry, etc.)

_____ how to tie knots

_____ horticulture

_____ animal husbandry

_____ tanning and leatherworking

_____ how to spin thread and weave cloth

_____ knitting, crocheting, and other needlework

_____ how to preserve food by drying, canning, pickling, etc.

_____ survival cookbook

_____ household hints, i.e., ways to substitute everyday items

Chapter 9

Maintenance Plan

Once you've laid out your plans, gathered supplies, and enhanced your dwelling, create a schedule to maintain your readiness. Conduct regular drills to practice your emergency procedures. Make it a game! Try to beat your time from the drill before.

MONTHLY

❑ Rotate your stock. If you regularly consume and replace your stock, very few perishables will have to be discarded. Check the following for freshness in your shelter, your vehicles, and at work:
  ❑ water
  ❑ food
  ❑ medicine
  ❑ batteries

❑ Perform routine maintenance on your vehicles.
  ❑ Check windshield-wiper fluid.
  ❑ Check radiator fluid.
  ❑ Check transmission fluid.
  ❑ Check power steering fluid.
  ❑ Check brake fluid.
  ❑ Check oil.
  ❑ Check belts.
  ❑ Check hoses.
  ❑ Check air filters.
  ❑ Check tires for air pressure and wear.
  ❑ Perform an alignment, if necessary.
  ❑ Perform a tune-up, if necessary.

❑ Inspect and test alarms.

❑ Conduct at least one of the following drills on a rotating basis:

  ❑ Conduct a fire drill: evacuate your home in the middle of the night. To simulate the smoky conditions you are likely to encounter in a fire, practice your evacuation drills blindfolded. See how long it takes everyone to reach your designated meeting place outside.

  ❑ Conduct a sheltering-in-place drill: get children and animals inside, fill sinks with water, turn off ventilation systems, and seal openings. See how long it takes everyone to reach their duty stations and perform their assigned tasks.

  ❑ Conduct an evacuation drill from home: evacuate your home within five minutes with three days of food. See how long it takes everyone to be in a vehicle and ready to roll. Drive on one of the evacuation routes out of your area. Take the route that you are least familiar with.

  ❑ Conduct an evacuation drill from work or school: walk from work to the nearest public shelter. If you have children, start from their schools and make them lead the way to the nearest public shelter. See how long it takes to reach a shelter, and determine where other shelters are located.

  ❑ Play "doctor." Practice taking blood pressure. giving CPR, applying pressure to a wound, splinting a broken limb, suturing (on an orange peel!), etc.

  ❑ Practice what to do if you are caught outside in a thunderstorm with no shelter nearby.

  ❑ Practice what to do if you are caught outside in a tornado or other high winds with no shelter nearby.

QUARTERLY

☐ Change the HEPA filters in your ventilation system.

☐ Change the clothing in your "go" bags to match the season. Replace clothing that has been outgrown.

☐ Check functionality of equipment and tools such as generators and sump pumps and perform maintenance and repairs as necessary.

☐ Clean up outside.

    ☐ Remove combustible materials, such as leaves, needles, and birds' nests, from the gutters and roof, especially at wall/roof intersections, in valleys, around vents, underneath tiles, around skylights, and from other nooks and crannies where embers could lodge themselves. Clear dead leaves, brush, and debris from around the house and deck. Clear debris from fences and walls.

    ☐ Trim back overgrown vegetation. Keep vegetation trimmed around windows and doors for greater visibility and added security. Trim vegetation around heater exhaust pipes and dryer vents to lessen the chance of fire. Trim branches close to windows to minimize breakage from high winds. Clear overhanging limbs from the perimeter of your home to keep the branches from falling under the weight of ice and snow onto your structure or power lines. Branches should be at least six feet from any structure.

☐ Check outside light bulbs and replace as necessary.

☐ Go camping or hiking to practice your survival skills.

☐ Learn something new. Take a class on plumbing, self-defense, navigation, or some other skill that you need to acquire.

SEMI-ANNUALLY

❑ Change batteries in smoke detectors.

❑ Inspect your roof each spring and fall for loose or missing shingles; repair or replace as needed.

ANNUALLY

❑ Inspect fire extinguishers and recharge as necessary.

❑ Check the supplies in your first aid kits. Replace perishables as necessary.

❑ Drain the waterbeds and refill with fresh water as necessary.

❑ Review your sheltering-in-place and evacuation plans to make sure they still meet your needs. Revise as necessary to add new family members or pets, or to account for a move to a new home or a new job, students away at school, or a change in health status.

❑ Review insurance coverage and update as necessary.

❑ Clean the chimney.

❑ Check weather-stripping on doors and windows, and seals on refrigerators and freezers. Replace as necessary.

❑ Disinfect your well, as appropriate.

❑ Pump out the septic tank, as appropriate.

❑ If you have a stream on your property, dredge the channel and shore up the levees, as necessary.

❑ Take a survival vacation. Go to a survival training school, or go primitive camping on your own.

Maintenance Plan
Monthly

❑ Rotate your stock.
❑ Perform routine maintenance on your vehicles.
❑ Inspect and test alarms.
❑ Conduct drills on a rotating basis.

Quarterly

❑ Change the HEPA filters in your ventilation system.
❑ Change the clothing in your "go" bags to match the season.
❑ Check functionality of equipment and tools.
❑ Clean up outside.
❑ Check outside light bulbs and replace as necessary.
❑ Go camping or hiking to practice your survival skills.
❑ Learn something new.

Semi-Annually

❑ Change batteries in smoke detectors.
❑ Inspect your roof for loose or missing shingles and repair as needed.

Annually

❑ Inspect fire extinguishers and recharge as necessary.
❑ Check the supplies in your first aid kits.
❑ Drain the waterbeds and refill with fresh water as necessary.
❑ Review your sheltering-in-place and evacuation plans to make sure they still meet your needs.
❑ Review insurance coverage and update as necessary.
❑ Clean the chimney.
❑ Check weather-stripping on doors and windows, and seals on refrigerators and freezers. Replace as necessary.
❑ Disinfect your well, as appropriate.
❑ Pump out the septic tank, as appropriate.
❑ If you have a stream on your property, dredge the channel and shore up the levees, as necessary.
❑ Take a survival vacation.

Section 2

During Disaster

This section details the ways to respond to emergencies as they occur.

This section has only one chapter. The first part of the chapter lists general responses that apply in all emergencies, and the remainder of the chapter lists responses that apply in specific kinds of emergencies.

Chapter 10

Responses To Disasters

Dangerous conditions can quickly escalate into life-threatening situations. One of the keys to survival is to pay attention to early warning signs and act right away. Sometimes clues to a looming disaster are present, such as the greenish storm clouds of an impending tornado or the hissing that precedes a gas-pipe explosion, but we choose to ignore them or downplay their significance. Notice how animals react when a storm is approaching. They don't know whether a storm is going to be mild or severe, they just know to take cover. Follow their lead. If you take precautions but the danger passes without incident, so what? It's better to be over-prepared than under-prepared.

In the midst of any disaster, if trained emergency personnel are present, follow their instructions. If trained emergency personnel are unavailable, put your own plans into action.

In many emergencies, your instinct will be to collect your children from school and meet other family members at home. If you have prepared your home well as an emergency shelter, it may be the safest place for you. However, depending on the type of disaster, the authorities may restrict travel, so you may have to wait to connect with other family members. In addition, if your home is in close proximity to the site of the disaster, your home may not be the safest place, in which case you must be prepared to evacuate with your survival kit.

In the case of an extreme catastrophe, you may disagree with authorities about the best course of action to take. The authorities may be telling everyone to remain where they are but you want to leave, or they may be telling everyone to evacuate but you want to stay. In some cases you may have the option to stay or to go, but if the authorities have declared a "state of emergency" or martial law, you will be required to follow their directives. To defy their orders will be an act of civil disobedience, and you will be subject to arrest. You will have to assess the risks and decide for yourself what is best. If the government loses control of the situation and anarchy ensues, you will be on your own.

SHORT WARNING

You have two choices: ride it out where you are, or try to escape. Remember that sometimes disasters are compounded by one another. As you consider your choices, think about the long-term consequences as well as the immediate effects of an event. For example, an ice storm not only makes roads hazardous immediately, it can also bring down power lines and cause a blackout that may last days or weeks. Should you stay or should you go? Consider these factors:

♦ Are you at work, at home, or somewhere else? Do you have time to safely reach the other members of your group?

♦ How well prepared is your home? If your emergency preparedness consists of a few cans of beans sitting in your pantry, you are ill-prepared; head for the nearest public shelter. If you have lots of water and food, a generator, and plenty of fuel, you may be able to ride out many disasters. However, you must consider other factors as well.

♦ How soon will the event arrive? A hurricane is usually tracked over water for several days before it makes landfall; you generally have sufficient time to either evacuate or board up your shelter to stay. On the other hand, when a tornado's funnel cloud appears, you don't have time to run from it; you must seek shelter immediately and ride it out.

♦ How soon will evacuation routes be affected? If you live in an urban area, evacuation routes will quickly become choked with traffic. If you live near a volcano, lava flows can cut off your evacuation route. Regardless of where you live, heavy rains and flooding can cause landslides and take out roads, bridges, and tunnels. If you need to leave to be safe, it's imperative to leave early and quickly.

♦ How severe is the event expected to be? If a nearby river is expected to overflow its banks and turn your front yard into a swamp, it might be worth the risk to stay. But if a large dam upstream breaks and unleashes a torrent of water that is expected to damage sewage treatment plants, gas lines, and power lines, as well as turn your living room into an aquarium, maybe it would be better to pack up and leave.

♦ How long is the danger expected to last? Can you afford to miss a lot of work? Can you afford to miss appointments?

NO WARNING

In a sudden survival situation, take immediate action:
- ❑ Call 911.
- ❑ Account for survivors.
- ❑ Administer first aid.
- ❑ Gather supplies and equipment.
- ❑ Seek shelter.
- ❑ Calm down, rest, and gather your wits. Assess your situation.
- ❑ Find warmth.
- ❑ Find water.
- ❑ Find food.

As you assess your situation, you have two options: stay where you are and wait for rescue, or leave, either to search for help or to get out on your own. Should you wait for rescue or leave on your own?

- ♦ What are the environmental conditions now, and how are they likely to change within the next few minutes, hours, or days? Is it going to get colder or hotter? Is it going to get wetter or drier? Is your exposure to biological toxins, hazardous chemicals, or radioactive fallout likely to increase?
- ♦ Do you have shelter or a way to build something?
- ♦ Do you have a way to stay warm? Do you have appropriate clothing? Do you have a way to build a fire?
- ♦ Do you have water and food or the means to obtain them?
- ♦ What other supplies do you have? What can you obtain on your own?
- ♦ Are you or others ill or injured? Are all of you able to travel?
- ♦ Do you have any means of communication (cell phone with service, flares, the ability to build a fire and send smoke signals, etc.)?
- ♦ Do you have any means of transportation?
- ♦ Do you know where you are? Do you know which direction to head? Are you on or near a busy route where you are likely to find help?
- ♦ Does anyone else know where you are? How long will it be before you are missed and someone comes looking for you?
- ♦ Who has the resources to help you? Are emergency personnel already overwhelmed? Are you just one of hundreds, or thousands, or millions who needs help?

EVACUATION

♦ Try to confine the disaster, if you have time to do so safely. Close openings, shut off ventilation systems, close tank valves, extinguish open flames, etc.

♦ Evacuate as quickly as possible, taking one of your planned escape routes.

♦ Leave your belongings behind. Do not carry any items with you (handbag, laptop, briefcase, etc.) as they will impede your travel.

♦ If you encounter smoke or vapor that is rising, stay low to the floor; crawl if you have to. If possible, cover your mouth and nose with a damp cloth.

♦ If you encounter vapor that is sinking, try to stay above it; walk on furniture if you have to. If possible, cover your mouth and nose with a damp cloth.

♦ Use stairs, not elevators.

♦ In a multi-story building, always go down to reach the ground level; never go up to reach the roof.

♦ If you are trapped in the building, try to make your way to a stairwell as a safe place to await rescue. Stairwells are designated exit routes and have fire-rated doors, concrete floors, and lighting.

♦ If you are trapped inside and cannot get to a stairwell, signal for help at a window. If you are above the second story, wait for rescue. Do not jump unless you are instructed to do so by trained emergency personnel.

♦ Help the deaf, blind, and disabled.

- In case of fire, feel doors before opening them.

  - If a door is hot, don't open it. If possible, use your alternate escape route. If you cannot leave the room, block off the vents and the bottom of the door to keep smoke out. Close all windows. Phone for help.

  - If a door is cool to the touch, open it slowly and proceed with caution. Close interior doors behind you, but don't lock them.

- Once you are outside, think "**UP**." Stay **uphill, upwind**, and **upstream** of the incident.

  Avoid traveling downwind or downstream from the disaster.

  - If you are at the site of the disaster, travel upwind.

  - If you are already upwind of the disaster, stay upwind.

  - If you are downwind of the disaster, travel across the wind.

- Call your local and long-distance contacts to report where you are going.

Pets

- Never leave pets or livestock behind in a locked area unless allowing them to roam would compromise their safety even more. If you can't take them with you, set them free so they can try to survive on their own.

- When you are traveling with pets, keep them on a leash or in a carrier.

Evacuation From Home

♦ If not all members of your group are present when you depart, leave a note telling the others when you left and where you are going.

♦ If you have time, shut off utilities before leaving your home if gas lines or water lines may be damaged.

    ♦ Shut off electricity to avoid potential fires. Turn off individual circuits first, then turn off the main circuit.

    ♦ Shut off natural gas to avoid potential fires.

    ♦ Shut off water at the main valve to avoid potential contamination from polluted waters.

    ♦ If utility service is not expected to be damaged, leave the utilities on to avoid losing the food in your refrigerator and freezer.

♦ If you have time, seal the house if biological, chemical, or radiological contamination is likely to occur.

♦ Lock your outside doors when leaving your home.

♦ If you have time, mark your home to let rescuers know that it is unoccupied by placing a large "X" next to the door using International Orange spray paint. Otherwise, they will break in to check for survivors.

Evacuation From Work

♦ If you have been instructed to do so, shut down equipment, as long as you will still have enough time to get out safely.

♦ Sound the alarms. This may include making an announcement over the intercom, pulling a fire alarm, or calling 911.

♦ Help others who need assistance, but only if you won't be putting yourself in danger. Leave difficult rescues to professionals.

♦ Report to your assigned assembly point so you can be accounted for.

Evacuation From Mass Transportation–Buses/Trains/Planes/Ships

♦ Follow the instructions of crew members; they are trained to assist you.

♦ Find the closest exit, which may be behind you. Escape hatches may also be in the ceiling or floor of buses and trains.

♦ If the aisle is blocked, climb over the seats.

♦ If exiting through smoke, stay close to the floor and cover your nose and mouth with fabric (shirt, jacket, or pillowcase), wet if possible.

♦ If you become involved in an emergency aboard a subway or above-ground train, get off at the next stop and do not linger. Leave the station immediately, going uphill and against the wind, if possible.

♦ In most circumstances, you should not leave a subway train that is between stations. The third rail may still be electrified, and trains may be running on adjacent tracks. Also be aware of overhead power lines; if they are touching the ground, it is not safe to leave the train. If you must leave a subway train between stations:

♦ Do not touch tracks or cables. You could be electrocuted.

♦ Use catwalks to exit the tunnel, if possible.

♦ Look for an emergency exit between stations. If none is available, continue carefully to the closest station.

♦ Once you reach the station, do not linger. Leave the area immediately, going uphill and against the wind, if possible.

♦ A subway or train emergency brake is intended to stop a runaway car. Pulling the emergency brake in any other situation is usually not recommended, as the cars will immediately stop where they are, and the brakes will have to be reset before the train can move again. Thus, if you are a long distance from the closest station, it will take rescuers longer to reach you. The emergency brake should only be used when forward momentum presents an imminent danger.

♦ In a plane, follow the white lights along the aisle to the red exit lights.

♦ If abandoning ship, put on a life jacket and move to the life rafts as quickly as possible.

♦ Once you are away from the vehicle or vessel, get as far away as possible to protect yourself from fire or an explosion.

TRANSPORTATION

The recommended course of action is to follow evacuation routes specified by authorities, since alternate routes may be dangerous or impassable. However, if the suggested roads become choked with fleeing traffic, it may be better to go a different way. Use any thoroughfare available. Use secondary streets, alleys, country roads, hiking trails, or bike paths. Take whatever avenue offers you and your family the best chance of survival.

If you have no other choice, you may be able to use the storm drain system to get out of town. ☠ **Warning:**

- **Use storm drains only if the chance of flooding is ZERO.** Do not enter storm drains if you are trying to escape a hurricane, a tornado, a broken dam, or any other water emergency that is going to dump a large volume of water into the drainage system.

- If it is a combined sewer system, the pipes carry both raw sewage and rain runoff. Stay out of these drain pipes, as the risk of infection is high.

- You may encounter homeless people living in the storm drains. The homeless aren't bad people, but some of them may be mentally unstable, and they are probably more street savvy than you are, so approach them with caution.

SHELTER

If you are at home, at work, or someplace else inside when disaster strikes, you may be able to remain there. If the structure isn't safe to stay in, you'll have to get out and seek shelter elsewhere. Or if you are outside when disaster strikes, you'll have to seek shelter. Whatever your situation is, you must find shelter before nightfall. Even in the desert, it gets chilly at night. If dusk is approaching, you'll have to act quickly.

The temperature tolerance range for humans is roughly mid-70's to upper 80's (degrees Fahrenheit). Within this thermal neutral zone, the human body is capable of regulating its core temperature to sustain life. Below 75 or above 87, the human body has to go into overdrive to protect itself from freezing or overheating, and this burns up a lot of calories. If the temperature is a lot below 75 or a lot above 87, your body won't be able to keep up and you'll die. This is why having a shelter is critical to your survival.

In most disaster situations, you need only temporary shelter, either because the event has a short timescale, or you expect to be rescued, or you will be moving to permanent quarters.

During Disaster

Shelter-in-place At Home

Depending on the nature of the disaster, do the following if you are sheltering-in-place at home:

♦ Fill up the kitchen sink, bathroom sinks, bathtubs, utility sink, clothes washer, and any other available container with water.

♦ Turn off ventilation systems in your shelter.

  ♦ forced-air heating systems
  ♦ air conditioners
  ♦ fans
  ♦ bathroom exhaust fans
  ♦ kitchen exhaust fans

♦ Seal openings with duct tape and plastic sheeting, allowing enough ventilation to prevent suffocation:

  ♦ windows
  ♦ doors
  ♦ fireplace dampers
  ♦ range or stove vents
  ♦ clothes dryer vents

♦ Strip and decontaminate children before entering your shelter.

♦ Decontaminate animals and herd them inside.

♦ If it is not safe to be above ground, stay in the basement. If it is not safe to be above ground and you don't have a basement, stay in the middle of the structure, as far as possible away from the windows.

♦ Take care of yourself first so you will be in a position to help other family members who need assistance.

♦ Be prepared to evacuate.

Shelter-In-Place Away From Home

If you are in an urban area, try to find a structure that is safe. This may be a designated public emergency shelter, or any other building, such as a hotel, a grocery store, or the lobby of an apartment building. If buildings aren't safe, try a bus or other vehicle.

If you are in a rural area and lucky enough to have a tent with you, you only need to pick a site. In choosing a site, consider the following:

Animals – Pick a site away from trails, away from animal tracks, and away from rocks or other crevices where reptiles and rodents live. Keep your tent closed so animals can't get in.

Falling Objects – Check overhead for loose-hanging limbs.

Run-off – Pick a site away from a sloping rock shelf to avoid water run-off, and away from any dirt banks to avoid mudslides.

Wind – Pick a site where you will be sheltered from the wind.

If you don't have a tent or other shelter materials with you, consider the natural elements in your environment that you can use as a "hasty" shelter: a cave, a rock overhang, a small clearing in the middle of a thicket, a fallen tree, or a hollow stump. Look for resident wildlife before moving in.

If you have to make your own shelter, see what materials are available.

- Make a simple lean-to by gathering dead limbs to make a frame, and lash them together with vines, shoe laces, or whatever you have. Cover the frame with leafy branches, evergreen boughs, or other plant material.
- Gather rocks and pile them up to build a protective wall.
- Burrow into a snow bank to make your own cave.

Avoid sleeping on the ground, since this can lower your body temperature to dangerous levels. Try one of these alternatives:

- If you don't have an air mattress or foam pad, sleep on a slab of bark or a layer of evergreen boughs to insulate you from the earth.
- If you have a large piece of material, use it to make a hammock to get you up off the ground, and build your shelter over it.
- Sleep in a tree on branches sturdy enough to support your weight.

FIREMAKING

Fire provides:
- warmth
- light
- a way to cook food
- safety from predators

How To Prepare Site

- Contain the fire so it doesn't burn out of control.
    - Dig a pit where the blaze will be. Clear the area around the pit of leaves, wood, and other flammable materials.
    - Surround the pit with a ring of rocks, if possible.
    - Make sure no overhanging branches will be too close to the flames.
- Keep your gear away from the pit.
- Keep tools nearby for extinguishing the flames in a hurry, such as a bucket of water or a shovel for throwing dirt or snow on the flames.
- If you want to hide your location, heavy tree cover and dense underbrush in the surrounding area can help to dissipate the smoke.
- If you want to reveal your location (to members of your group, other friendly camps, or rescuers, for example), burn in a clearing where smoke can rise and be seen. Also burn green wood, which makes more smoke than seasoned wood.
- Make a reflector to radiate heat towards your body. Place a sheet of metal or a wall of rocks behind the fire.

How To Start A Fire

- cigarette lighter
- matches
- metal match or flint and steel
- steel wool and a battery
- shiny metal to reflect energy from the sun onto the tinder
- friction using a hand drill, bow drill, pump drill, or similar device

How To Build A Fire

Tinder – the smallest pieces, such as dried grass, leaves, small twigs
Kindling – the middle–sized pieces, such as small branches
Fuel – the largest pieces, such as split logs

♦ Start with the tinder, add kindling, and then add fuel, in that order. Give each stage time to burn and to ignite the next biggest pieces of wood.
♦ A fire must have air to burn. Arrange the material loosely.
♦ Wood must be dry to burn. A piece of kindling snaps when dry but bends when wet. Tap a log with a rock or branch; if it makes a clear knocking sound, it is dry; if it sounds like a dull thud, it is wet.
♦ Bark insulates the wood and makes it difficult to burn. Split the logs with an ax or sharp stone to expose the heart of the wood for easier burning.

How To Maintain A Fire

♦ Softwoods (conifers, i.e., evergreens, such as pine and cedar) ignite easily and burn quickly.
♦ Hardwoods (deciduous trees, i.e., broadleaf trees that lose their leaves, such as oak, maple, birch, cherry, and walnut) are harder to ignite and burn slowly.
♦ If you have a choice of both kinds of wood, use softwoods for tinder and kindling to get the fire started and building rapidly, and then use hardwoods to keep the fire going for a long time.
♦ Keep the fire going by periodically adding logs to the fire.
♦ Cook food with coals. Coals allow you to control the cooking process easier than flames.

How To Extinguish A Fire

♦ Allow the flames to die down and cover the coals with dirt. Use this method if you expect to restart the fire in the same place later.
♦ Pour a bucket of water on the flames, and then cover with dirt. Use this method if you will be moving on.

How To Restart A Fire

♦ Dig out a shovel-full of hot coals from the dirt. Once exposed to the air, add some tinder and kindling to restart the blaze.

WATER

Minimize the amount of water your body needs by reducing your activity level and staying cool in hot weather.

Stored Water

If you are using home-bottled water, check it with the "smell" test. If the odor of chlorine is not detectable, treat the water with chlorine and allow it to sit for 30 minutes; repeat the process until a slight odor of chlorine is present. If possible, run the water through a carbon filter to remove TTHMs before drinking.

If power is available, store opened containers in a refrigerator at or below 40° Fahrenheit to retard the growth of bacteria.

Alternate Water Sources

Depending on the type of disaster, your water supply at home may not be affected immediately, but may become tainted later if damage has occurred to water or sewer lines or your local water treatment facility   At the beginning of an emergency, as long as you are confident that your water supply has not yet been contaminated, fill bathtubs and sinks with water. These containers can supplement the stored water that you have already stocked. Then shut off incoming water at the main valve into your home to prevent contaminated water from entering your pipes.

If your stored water supply runs low, you can use the following sources. Note that water from sources outside your piping system will have to be treated to be safe from chemical and biological contamination.

♦   ice cubes

♦   water pipes – Drain water from the pipes by turning on the faucets, starting with those at the highest level in your home.

♦   toilet tanks

- hot water tanks
    - Shut off power to the tank (electricity at the circuit breaker or gas at the pilot light).
    - Shut off the water intake valve.
    - Turn on a hot-water faucet somewhere in the house to prevent a vacuum in the lines.
    - Open the drain valve at the bottom of the tank and collect the water in a bucket, or attach a hose and run the water wherever you like.
    - Do not use this water if the water tank or other plumbing fixtures are submerged by flood.
    - Do not turn on gas or electricity to the tank when it is empty.

- waterbed
    - Use this water only if it has been treated to remove chemicals and microorganisms.
    - Use this water only for showering or flushing toilets.

- hot tub or pool
    - Use this water only if it has been treated to remove chemicals and microorganisms.
    - Use this water only for showering or flushing toilets.

- moving water from streams and rivers
    - Use this water only if it has been treated to remove chemicals and microorganisms.

- standing water from ponds and lakes
    - Use this water only if it has been treated to remove chemicals and microorganisms.

- rainwater

- dew

- plant stalks

Water from a well or spring is usually safe to drink. If you have any doubts, treat it with iodine or chlorine.

All surface water, whether moving or still, should be considered contaminated and will have to be treated.

Water Treatment

Tainted water needs to be purified by removing or killing biological contaminants, removing chemical contaminants, and/or removing radiological contaminants. Purification can be accomplished by filtration, heat sterilization, ultraviolet radiation, solar disinfection, chemical disinfection, distillation, reverse osmosis, and desalination. (See Chapter 4 for more information on these methods.) The method to use depends on the kind of contaminants you are trying to eliminate and the resources you have available.

If you have limited resources, perform as many of the following steps as possible:

1. Remove debris.

    a. Strain water through layers of clean cloth (towel, sheet, shirt, etc.) or paper (coffee filter, paper towel, etc.).

    b. If you don't have a way to strain the water, allow enough time to let suspended particles settle to the bottom.

2. Eliminate biological, chemical, and radiological contaminants using:

    a. a reverse osmosis system coupled with a carbon filter, or

    b. a distillation system coupled with a carbon filter

3. If you do not have access to a reverse osmosis system or a distillation system:

    a. Eliminate biological contaminants using one of the following:

> heat
> UV radiation
> solar disinfection
> iodine
> chlorine

    b. Eliminate chemical contaminants using a carbon filter.

FOOD

Healthy adults can live without any food for several days, and can subsist on half their normal caloric intake for many days or even weeks.

Growing children, pregnant women, nursing mothers, and the sick should receive regular balanced meals to meet their nutritional needs, so if you don't have enough food to go around, feed these group members first.

Use food with the shortest shelf-life first. Use your food in this order:

1. Perishables from the refrigerator and garden

2. Perishables from the freezer

3. Non-perishables from the pantry

When the power goes out, food in your freezer will remain usable for 24 - 48 hours if you don't open the door.

Do not take food from outside into your shelter if there is any possibility it is contaminated by a biological agent, a chemical agent, or radiation. Rely on your stored goods.

Alternate Food Sources

If you have to trap, hunt, fish, or forage for food in the wild, refer to the survival manuals and field guides in your library for help.

Alternate Cooking Methods

♦ Cook directly on a heated stone.

♦ Drop hot rocks into a pot to cook the food in the pot.

♦ Wrap food in aluminum foil, tree leaves, or corn husks and cook directly on top of the coals.

♦ Three-stone cooking fire – Three flat stones of the same height are placed in a triangle around the fire and a cooking pot is set on the stones over the fire.

♦ Two logs can be placed parallel with the fire in the middle and a cooking pot is set on top of the logs.

♦ Pots with legs, such as a Dutch oven, can be set over a fire.

♦ Pots with handles can be suspended over a fire, using a tripod, a crane, or a horizontal crosspiece between two vertical posts.

♦ Earth oven – dig a pit in the ground, throw in hot rocks or coals from the fire, add the food, cover with dirt; or use an existing fire pit, burn the fire down to embers, throw on the food, and cover with dirt.

ENERGY

If you are using a portable generator, lock and tag your main circuit breaker to the house to prevent backfeed. Use the interlock or transfer switch to allow your electrical panel to feed off the generator; otherwise, you will need several extension cords to run from the generator to various appliances in your home. Do NOT use an extension cord with two male ends, one to plug into the generator and one into an outlet, as this creates an electrical hazard.

☠ **Warning: To avoid carbon monoxide poisoning, never use gas-powered equipment in an attached garage or closed living space. Generators, portable grills, space heaters, or any other equipment or appliances powered by any kind of gas must be vented to the outside.**

☠ **Warning: If you are using a portable generator, turn off the main house breaker to prevent backfeed.**

☠ **Warning: Do not vent a solid-fuel appliance into a chimney that is used by a gas furnace or gas water heater. This is dangerous.**

Alternate Sources of Energy

♦ vehicle battery

♦ power outlets on cars, trucks, RV's, or boats

COMMUNICATIONS

You don't need an electrical cord, cable service, or satellite dish to find out what's going on. A battery-powered TV with an antenna can receive broadcast stations with news and updates.

Rely on the equipment and services still working: wire-based phone, cell phone, satellite phone, wire-based computer, battery-powered computer, hand-cranked radio, walkie-talkies, CB radio, etc.

If you are stranded aboard a watercraft or aircraft but you have radio communications, issue a pan-pan call or a mayday call.

▶ Three repetitions of "Pan-Pan" signify an urgency without immediate danger to life. The message would be:

> "Pan-Pan, Pan-Pan, Pan-Pan"
> "All Stations, All Stations, All Stations"
> Name of vessel or call sign
> Position of craft (latitude & longitude)
> Nature of problem
> Type of assistance required, if any

▶ Three repetitions of "Mayday" signify an emergency with imminent danger to life and are a request for immediate assistance. The message would be:

> "Mayday, Mayday, Mayday"
> Name of vessel or call sign, given 3 times
> "Mayday"
> Name of vessel or call sign
> Position of craft (latitude & longitude)
> Nature of problem
> Type of assistance required

How to Attract Attention When Stranded

If you don't have a working cell phone or satellite phone or two-way radio, you will have to make contact with rescuers with a visual signal or one that is audible from a distance. Your signal must communicate two pieces of information: **notification of your emergency situation** and your **location.**

♦ Set off flares, but only if you're sure they are within range of being seen.

♦ Build a fire in an open area as high up as possible. Create smoke by burning grass, leaves, green sticks, tires, or whatever is available.

♦ Lay out rocks, logs, or other vegetation in a large formation that can be seen from the sky: X or SOS. Or stamp SOS into a snow bank.

♦ Signal SOS with a mirror or flashlight (3 short flashes, 3 long flashes, 3 short flashes).

♦ Signal SOS with a horn (3 short blasts, 3 long blasts, 3 short blasts).

♦ Display signals in groups of three: three piles of rocks, three fires, three of whatever you have available.

♦ Display signal flags "N" and "C" together to indicate distress ("N" is a blue and white checkerboard pattern; "C" is a pattern of horizontal stripes in blue-white-red-white-blue). The "N" flag represents the word "no" or "negative." The "C" flag represents the word "yes" or "affirmative." Displaying these two flags together is an international distress signal.

♦ Display a square flag with a ball or other circular object above or below it.

♦ Attract attention by creating an unusual visual display, such as hoisting a jib sail upside down, flying a flag upside down, flying a flag with a knot in it, etc.

♦ If a vehicle, aircraft, or watercraft is in sight, raise both arms at an angle to indicate "Y," as in "Yes, I need help," or wave both arms above your head.

Assault

♦ Avoid confrontation if possible. Don't do anything to provoke an attack, even if you are "right" and the other person is "wrong."

♦ If you are forced to resist, end the altercation as quickly as possible and retreat. In a survival situation, the goal is not to "win" the fight. The goal is to minimize your injuries and improve your odds of survival.

♦ If someone attacks you, scream or blow a whistle to attract attention. Yell "This person is a stranger!" Teach your children to yell "This is not my parent!"

♦ Look for something you can use as a weapon. A weapon can be anything that gives you an advantage or places your adversary at a disadvantage.
  ♦ natural materials, such as a stick, a log, a stone, or dirt that you can throw in the eyes
  ♦ a piece of glass or pottery
  ♦ construction materials, such as a brick, a board, or a piece of pipe
  ♦ tools, such as a shovel, a tire iron, a hammer, or a screwdriver
  ♦ sports equipment, such as a golf club, a baseball bat, or an oar

♦ If someone in a car harasses you while you are walking, turn around and walk the other way. Go to a nearby business or other public facility.

♦ If you see a baby seat in the road, or if objects are thrown at your vehicle, don't stop, as it is probably a ploy to get you to park your vehicle and put you in a vulnerable position. Instead, continue a safe distance and call 911.

♦ If you break down on the road, call a towing service or 911 for help. If someone stops and offers you a ride, decline it and ask them to summon the police for you. Never get into a stranger's vehicle.

♦ If someone tries to force your vehicle off the road, put the car in reverse and back away. Honk the horn to attract attention.

- Criminals may intentionally cause a vehicle accident, either to file a false insurance claim, extort money from you, or rob you. If you are involved in a fender bender that seems suspicious, or if you feel uncomfortable about the circumstances, do not get out of your vehicle. Instead, stay in your vehicle and call 911 immediately. If you feel threatened, leave the scene and call 911 immediately.

- If an attacker tries to force you into a vehicle, do everything in your power to resist. Let them have everything – your keys, your car, your money, your credit cards, your jewelry – but do not get into the vehicle.

- If you think someone is following you, go to a police station, a fire station, or a public place such as a retail store or other business where other people are around. Do not lead the pursuer to your home.

- If you live in an apartment building, don't give strangers access to your building. If strangers ask to be let in, tell them to contact the resident they wish to visit, or offer to contact the resident for them.

- If you are the first person to arrive home and your entry door is not locked, don't go inside. Call the police from your cell phone, a neighbor's home, or a nearby business.

- Do not let strangers into your home. If strangers knock on your door and ask to use the phone in an emergency, make them stay outside and tell them that you will call emergency services for them.

- Service technicians always wear uniforms and always display a photo ID badge. If you have scheduled service technicians to come to your home, make sure they are wearing uniforms and ID badges before you let them in. If you have not scheduled any service and technicians show up on your doorstep "just to check things out," do not let them in. If they offer you a phone number to call to verify their identity, do not use it, as the person who answers the phone may be part of the deception. Instead, call the number on your billing statement to verify the unscheduled activity and confirm the badge numbers.

During Disaster

Avalanche

Rescue Yourself

♦ If you're buried beneath the surface, punch out an area of the snow around you to make an air pocket. Take a deep breath and hold it to expand your chest; otherwise, once the snow sets, you may not be able to breathe. Act quickly, because once the avalanche stops, you will have only a few seconds until the snow sets.

Rescue Another

♦ If you are alone, don't see any signs of the victim, and don't have a transceiver, go for help.

♦ If you are with another person, one of you should go for help while the other looks for the victim. To search for the victim:

  ♦ Turn your transceiver to receive signals.
  ♦ Look for arms, legs, ski poles, gloves, or anything else that might indicate where the victim is. If you don't see any signs of the victim, work your way along the avalanche path. If you are above the victim, start at the place where you last saw the victim and work your way down the slope to the run-out zone where the snow comes to rest. If you are below the victim, work your way back up the slope. Concentrate on areas where the snow and debris have piled up, such as the uphill side of trees and the outside edge of turns.
  ♦ Remember that snowmobilers are usually located uphill of their snowmobiles.
  ♦ To cover the widest range possible, probe to the right, probe to the center, and probe to the left. If you don't have an avalanche probe, use a tree branch.

Biological Incident

A biological disaster:

- involves organisms that harm or kill crops, animals, or people
- may be caused by bacteria, viruses, or toxins
- may be caused by natural forces, such as an invasion of killer bees or a naturally spreading epidemic, or it may be caused by humans, either accidentally, such as an unintended release from a research facility, or deliberately, such as an attack by terrorists
- may be delivered through food and water supplies or by airborne sprays, weapons, or animals, including insects and humans
- contamination may be contracted by:
    - inhaling contaminated air
    - ingesting contaminated food or water
    - insect or animal bites or other contact with contaminated animals or animal products
    - contact with an affected individual: skin, mucous membranes (mouth, nose, eyes), other body orifices (ears, genitals, anus)
    - contact with contaminated soil

Clues: Indications of a Possible Biological Incident

- discarded spray devices
- unusual aerial spraying
- dead animals, including mammals, birds, reptiles, insects, fish (manifestations may range from hours to years)
- mass human casualties: unusually high number of individuals exhibiting similar unexplained symptoms, becoming sick, or dying (manifestations may range from hours to years)

During Disaster

At Home

♦ Remove contaminated clothing.
♦ Wash with antibacterial soap or a waterless antibacterial solution.
♦ Line-drying clothes in the sun kills anthrax spores by exposing them to ultraviolet rays. (Alcohol is ineffective against anthrax spores.)
♦ Get inside with children and pets.
♦ Close and lock all outside doors, windows and vents.
♦ Unpack your plastic sheeting to cover the openings of your shelter. Using duct tape, secure each plastic sheet at the corners, and then seal the edges. Cover all doors, windows, and vents. At the bottom edges of doors, extend the plastic a few inches into the room at a right angle over the floor to make sure the gap between the door and the threshold is sealed off.
♦ If you don't have plastic sheeting, close the draperies, curtains, blinds, or shades.
♦ Stay in an interior room (i.e., one without windows) above ground level (biological agents are usually heavier than air and will sink to ground level).
♦ Listen to the radio or TV or access the Internet for updates on what areas have been exposed, what symptoms to watch for, and what to do if you think you have been infected.
♦ Avoid going out in public. If you must go out in public, wear gloves and a mask.
♦ Avoid eating at public establishments.
♦ If you become sick, seek medical attention as soon as possible.
♦ Consider vaccination if a vaccine is available.
♦ Be prepared to be quarantined.
♦ Be prepared to evacuate.

In a Vehicle

♦ Pull to the side of the road or the safest place possible.
♦ Turn off the engine.
♦ Turn off heater or air conditioner.
♦ Close the windows and vents. Seal the vents with plastic and duct tape.
♦ Listen to the radio for updates from the authorities.
♦ When ready to travel, head upwind or crosswind from the release site.

In Public

◆ Try not to inhale. Hold your breath as long as possible until you get out of the immediate vicinity of the release; when you must breathe, take shallow breaths.

◆ Cover you nose and mouth with a respirator, mask, or several layers of fabric (wet if possible). If you don't have fabric, use layers of tissue or paper towels.

◆ Keep your eyes closed as much as possible, as long as it does not inhibit escape.

◆ Do not touch your eyes, nose, or mouth.

◆ Cover exposed skin.

◆ If instructed by emergency personnel to stay in place for decontamination, you should do so. Otherwise, leave the area of exposure immediately.

◆ Travel in a direction that will lead you away from the site of the disaster, against the wind and uphill, if possible.

  ◆ Travel on foot.

  ◆ If you take your own vehicle, you may contaminate it, and it will have to be decontaminated later. On the other hand, if you believe you will have to abandon the vehicle later anyway, it doesn't matter if it becomes contaminated.

  ◆ Avoid mass transit. Public transportation will quickly become overwhelmed, and the more people you are around, the greater your chances of contamination.

◆ Do not touch suspicious substances, packages, or containers.

◆ Seek shelter. If an explosion has taken place, make sure the building you choose is not in imminent danger of collapsing.

During Disaster

♦ Once you reach shelter, remove your clothes and seal them in plastic bags. If possible, remove clothes outside; do not take them into your shelter.

♦ Wash intact skin with antimicrobial soap and hot running water, or a waterless antibacterial solution.

♦ Broken skin should be encouraged to bleed; then the wound should be cleaned and dressed.

♦ Flush eyes with saline solution or plain water.

♦ Seek medical treatment if necessary.

♦ Stay inside your shelter with the doors and windows sealed. If you must go outside, wear a mask and other protective clothing. Facial hair reduces the effectiveness of respiratory masks. Shave!

♦ Listen to the TV or radio for updated information from authorities. Once authorities have identified the nature of the attack, follow their instructions on medical treatment and environmental decontamination.

♦ Avoid close physical contact with others.

♦ Wash your clothes and bedding in disinfectant and hot water.

♦ Clean surfaces, especially in the kitchen, with disinfectant and hot water.

♦ If treating a sick member of your group who may have a communicable disease, wear a disposable mask, gown, and gloves.

Children

♦ Check children for scrapes and scratches that would allow bacteria or viruses to enter the bloodstream.

♦ Closely monitor children who have been exposed to a biological agent. They are more susceptible to illness because their immune systems are not fully developed. In addition, children breathe faster than adults, so for their body size, they inhale relatively greater doses of a biological agent than an adult does. Check for any signs of a developing illness, such as coughing, difficulty breathing, sluggishness, fever, or rash.

♦ Children are more likely than adults to become dehydrated from vomiting and diarrhea. If they experience these symptoms, be sure they receive plenty of fluids.

Pets

♦ Like people, pets should not go outside during biological emergencies.

♦ If pets may be contaminated, they should be washed thoroughly with soap and water before bringing them inside your shelter.

♦ If you are evacuating, your pets will be safest evacuating, too. You have no guarantee of when, if ever, you will be able to return home.

Blackout/Brownout

A "blackout" is a total loss of electric power. A "brownout" is a lowering of voltage for an extended period of time, causing lights to flicker, motor-driven appliances to falter, and computers to crash. Blackouts and brownouts may be due to a mechanical failure, a supply shortage resulting from consumer demand, or a terrorist attack on the grid.

In the event of a blackout:

♦ Light candles, lanterns, etc. so you can see what you're doing.

♦ In cold temperatures, bring blankets out of storage.

♦ Start running your generator, but only for essential services, such as operating a refrigerator or freezer, operating a well pump, operating a space heater, etc.

♦ If you don't have a generator to keep food cold, tape a sign to the refrigerator and freezer to remind everyone not to open the doors.

Blizzard

♦ Stay inside. However tempting it may be for kids to go out and make snow angels or play in the falling snow, use caution. Those blowing winds - both before and after a blizzard - are cold enough to cause frostbite, and snowdrifts may hide dangers that children might otherwise see.

♦ If you are on the road when a blizzard hits, look for a hotel and stay off the roads until driving conditions are safe again.

♦ If you become stranded in your vehicle during a storm:

  ♦ Get your emergency supplies out of the trunk.

  ♦ Tie a flag or piece of cloth to your antenna to signal that you are in distress. If it's not snowing, also raise the hood to signal for help.

  ♦ Wrap yourself in blankets and extra clothing to stay warm.

  ♦ Move your arms and legs to improve circulation and stay warm.

  ♦ Huddle with other passengers to stay warm.

  ♦ Run the engine and heater in short bursts (about 10 minutes every hour), just long enough to get the vehicle warm and then turn it off. Keep one window open just a little to avoid carbon monoxide poisoning. Do not run the engine continuously to keep warm, because the danger of carbon monoxide poisoning is high. Snow can block your exhaust pipe and fill the car with deadly fumes. In addition, if you keep the engine running continuously, you may run out of fuel before the storm is over.

  ♦ Try to stay awake so you can monitor your temperature.

  ♦ If you're thirsty, melt snow to bring it to a warmer temperature before drinking it. Eating snow will lower your body temperature.

  ♦ Stay with your vehicle and wait until help arrives or until conditions are stable enough for you to get back on the road.

Chemical Incident

Lethal chemical agents include:

♦ choking agents, also known as asphyxiants or respiratory agents; they affect your ability to breathe by burning lung tissue, also called "dry land drowning;" examples: chlorine gas or phosgene

♦ blister agents; they cause burns and blisters on skin and eyes; inhaling them can burn the throat and lungs and can be fatal; example: mustard gas

♦ blood agents; they prevent respiration on a cellular level; without oxygen reaching your cells, you'll suffocate; example: cyanide

♦ nerve agents; deadliest type of chemical agents; colorless and usually odorless; they act quickly and suffocate by paralyzing muscles in and around the lungs; example: sarin gas

Chemicals:

♦ may be dispersed accidentally, such as a spill from a train wreck or truck crash or an unintended release from a production facility, or deliberately, such as an attack by terrorists

♦ may be in the form of powder, liquid, or gas

♦ may be delivered through food and water supplies or by aerosol sprays or aerial sprayers, or by weapons or explosives, such as grenades, mines, or bombs

♦ may enter the body through:
  ♦ inhaling contaminated air
  ♦ ingesting contaminated food or water
  ♦ skin absorption

Clues: Indications of a Possible Chemical Incident

♦ unusual metal debris, left from detonation of bomb

♦ abandoned spray devices

♦ unusual aerial spraying

♦ hazy atmosphere, unexplained by weather or usual environmental conditions

♦ unexplained odors, out of character with surroundings

♦ unusual liquid droplets, such as oily droplets and an absence of recent rain

♦ dead vegetation, unexplained by weather or season

♦ dead animals, including mammals, birds, reptiles, insects, fish (manifestations may range from seconds to days)

♦ mass human casualties: unusually high number of individuals exhibiting similar unexplained symptoms, becoming sick, or dying (manifestations may range from seconds to days)

♦ casualties that occur within a confined geographic area

♦ casualties distributed in a pattern

♦ symptoms may include labored breathing, a burning sensation in the nose, throat, or lungs, eye irritation, nausea, and poor coordination

If you are exposed to a chemical:

♦ Cover your nose and mouth with paper or cloth. But don't use outer clothing that may be contaminated.

♦ If your eyes burn, remove contact lenses and flush your eyes with cool water from the nose outward.

♦ Remove your clothes, starting at the top. Avoid brushing the contaminated clothing against your skin.

♦ Place your clothing in a plastic bag.

♦ Wash your body with cool water, taking care not to scrub the chemical into your skin. If you're away from home, use a public restroom, a drinking fountain, a hose, or any source of water you can find.

♦ If water isn't available, close your eyes and brush the chemical off your skin.

♦ If the chemical has burned your skin, cover the wound loosely with a dry, sterile cloth and seek medical attention.

♦ Avoid touching others who have been contaminated. With chemical exposure, it's possible to be affected by touching a contaminated person.

♦ Call 911.

♦ Seek medical attention.

♦ If you ingest poison, call 911 or a poison control center. Do not induce vomiting unless advised to do so, since more damage may be done to the esophagus, throat or lungs.

At Home

♦ After removing contaminated clothing and washing off with water, get inside with children and pets.

♦ Close and lock all outside doors, windows and vents.

♦ Unpack your plastic sheeting to cover the openings of your shelter. Using duct tape, secure each plastic sheet at the corners, and then seal the edges. Cover all doors, windows, and vents. At the bottom edges of doors, extend the plastic a few inches into the room at a right angle over the floor to make sure the gap between the door and the threshold is sealed off.

♦ If you don't have plastic sheeting, close the draperies, curtains, blinds, or shades.

♦ Stay in an interior room (i.e., one without windows) above ground level (chemical agents are usually heavier than air and will sink to ground level).

♦ Listen to the radio or TV or access the Internet for updates on what areas have been exposed, what symptoms to watch for, and what to do if you think you have been exposed.

♦ Avoid going out in public. If you must go out in public, wear gloves and a mask.

♦ Avoid eating at public establishments.

♦ If you become sick, seek medical attention as soon as possible.

♦ Be prepared to evacuate.

In a Vehicle

♦ Pull to the side of the road or the safest place possible.

♦ Turn off the engine.

♦ Turn off heater or air conditioner.

♦ Close the windows and vents. Seal the vents with plastic and duct tape.

♦ Listen to the radio for updates from the authorities.

♦ When ready to travel, head upwind or crosswind from the release site.

In Public

♦ If a harmful chemical is released indoors, get out of the building as quickly as possible. If you can't get out of the building, get as far away as you can from the release site.

♦ If a harmful chemical is released outdoors and you are indoors, stay inside and seal the building. Be prepared to shelter-in-place as the chemical spreads.

♦ If you are in a multi-story building, go up to the higher floors. Chemical agents are usually heavier than air and will sink to ground level.

♦ If a harmful chemical is released outdoors and you are outdoors, get to clean air as quickly as possible. Leave the area immediately, if you can, heading upwind or crosswind from the release site. If you cannot leave the area, seek shelter inside a nearby building. Seal the building and be prepared to shelter-in-place as the chemical spreads.

♦ Try not to inhale. Hold your breath as long as possible until you get out of the immediate vicinity of the release; when you must breathe, take shallow breaths.

♦ Cover you nose and mouth with a respirator, mask, or several layers of fabric (wet if possible). If you don't have fabric, use layers of tissue or paper towels.

♦ Keep your eyes closed as much as possible, as long as it does not inhibit escape.

♦ Do not touch your eyes, nose, or mouth.

♦ Cover exposed skin.

♦ If instructed by emergency personnel to stay in place for treatment, you should do so. Otherwise, leave the area of exposure immediately.

- Travel in a direction that will lead you away from the site of the disaster, against the wind and uphill, if possible.

  - Travel on foot.
  - If you take your own vehicle, you may contaminate it, and it will have to be decontaminated later. On the other hand, if you believe you will have to abandon the vehicle later anyway, it doesn't matter if it becomes contaminated.
  - Avoid mass transit. Public transportation will quickly become overwhelmed, and the more people you are around, the greater your chances of contamination.

- Do not touch suspicious substances, packages, or containers.

- Seek shelter away from the release site. If you have been exposed to a chemical agent that is heavier than air, do not lie on the floor or go below ground. If an explosion has occurred, make sure the building you choose is not in imminent danger of collapsing.

- Once you reach shelter, remove your clothes and seal them in plastic bags. If possible, remove clothes outside; do not take them into your shelter.

- Wash intact skin with soap and hot running water.

- Broken skin should be encouraged to bleed; then the wound should be cleaned and dressed.

- Flush eyes with saline solution or plain water.

- Seek medical treatment if necessary.

- Stay inside your shelter with the doors and windows sealed. If you must go outside, wear a mask and other protective clothing. Facial hair reduces the effectiveness of respiratory masks. Shave!

- Listen to the TV or radio for updated information from authorities. Once authorities have identified the nature of the attack, follow their instructions on medical treatment and environmental decontamination.

- Avoid close physical contact with others.

During Disaster

Children

♦ Check children for scrapes and scratches that would allow toxins to enter the bloodstream.

♦ Closely monitor children who have been exposed to a chemical agent. If the chemicals used are heavier than air, children could be affected more, simply because they are closer to the ground. In addition, children breathe faster than adults, so for their body size, they inhale relatively greater doses of a chemical agent than an adult does. Furthermore, the skin of children is more permeable than that of adults, so agents that are absorbed through the skin would pose a greater danger to children. Check for complaints of burning eyes, nose, throat, or skin; excessive salivation or profuse mucus production in nasal passages and airways; choking or difficulty breathing; chest pain; nausea or vomiting; involuntary release of urine or stool; blisters, welts, or rashes; dilated pupils; changes in skin color; headache; blurred vision; dizziness, disorientation, or lack of coordination; trembling, convulsions, paralysis, or loss of consciousness.

♦ Children are more likely than adults to become dehydrated from vomiting and diarrhea. If they experience these symptoms, be sure they receive plenty of fluids.

Pets

♦ Like people, pets should not go outside during chemical emergencies.

♦ If pets may be contaminated, they should be washed thoroughly with soap and water before bringing them inside your shelter.

♦ If you are evacuating, your pets will be safest evacuating, too. You have no guarantee of when, if ever, you will be able to return home.

Civil Unrest

♦ If possible, withdraw from any area of civil unrest to avoid confrontations.

♦ Be wary of checkpoints and roadblocks during periods of lawlessness. They may be operated by "freelancers" who are trying to shake down innocent victims or detour them into a trap. Even at "legitimate" checkpoints, you may be interrogated or searched.

If you approach a checkpoint or roadblock, watch what happens to the people in front of you. If you don't like what you see, you can turn around. However, turning away will raise suspicion, and the operators of the checkpoint are likely to come after you for questioning anyway. If you are uncomfortable about passing through checkpoints and roadblocks, try to find out where they are and avoid them by taking an alternate route.

Cold

To survive, humans must maintain a body temperature close to 98°F. Staying warm is of more immediate importance than finding water or food.

To stay warm, minimize the loss of body heat and add heat through any means possible.

♦ Build a fire as soon as possible.

♦ Build a shelter as soon as possible.

♦ Huddle with a group of people or animals.

♦ Wear loose clothing. Tight-fitting clothing may restrict circulation.

♦ Dress in layers to trap body heat, using materials that allow perspiration to escape.

♦ Wear clothing made of wind-breaking material that also allows perspiration to escape.

♦ Remove wet clothing and put on dry clothing immediately. When moisture on your skin evaporates, body heat goes with it.

♦ Don't touch cold objects with your bare skin. Any time you touch something colder than your body, you lose body heat.

♦ Don't sleep directly on the ground. Use boughs, leaves, bark, grass, or whatever is available to insulate you from the earth.

- If you are sheltering outdoors, you can heat rocks in a fire and use them several ways to keep warm: (BEWARE! Rocks may contain water that causes them to explode when heated, so keep a safe distance from the fire when heating rocks.)

    - Dig a small pit in the dirt inside your shelter and toss the hot rocks into the pit to create a furnace.

    - Bury the hot rocks in the dirt under your sleeping bag for added warmth. Allow the steam to evaporate before placing your bag or mattress over the top of the trench or you'll get wet. Or instead of moving the rocks in and out of the fire, set them up as a lining to your fire pit. At bedtime, rake the coals out of the fire pit, cover the hot rocks with several inches of dirt, wait for the steam to escape, and then place your bedding on top.

    - If you let the hot rocks cool down a little, you can put them directly into your sleeping bag or bed instead of burying them.

- Heat beverages such as coffee, tea, or soup. Breathing the air across the top of the container warms the air before inhaling it into your lungs, and drinking the liquid warms your digestive tract.

- If you have plenty of food, warm up by working or exercising. Physical activity warms the body from the inside, but it also burns calories, which you will have to replenish with food. If you don't have much food, you can't afford to burn calories to stay warm.

- Heat water and fill a container with it. Place the container over your kidneys. As blood passes through your kidneys, it picks up heat and carries the warmth throughout your body.

Coronal Mass Ejection (CME)

A coronal mass ejection is the sun spewing charged particles into space. The sun does this sort of thing all the time; it's why we have the Northern Lights and the Southern Lights. A coronal mass ejection would be a problem for us only if we encountered an unusually large one.

The most likely effects would be:

♦ satellites knocked out of their orbits, thereby disrupting television and radio transmissions, credit card transactions, phone services, GPS systems, etc.

♦ a surge in electric current that could overload power grids and cause widespread blackouts

♦ radiation sickness for humans in space or in airplanes

If you lose some communications services, rely on the equipment and services still working: wire-based phone, a battery-powered TV with an antenna, battery-powered or hand-cranked radio, walkie-talkies, CB radio, ham radio, VHF radio, etc.

If you lose electric power, rely on your backup equipment: candles, lanterns, emergency generator, etc.

If you are exposed to radiation, create a barrier as thick as possible between you and the source of the radiation. Seek shelter underground. If you are in a public place, look for a yellow and black "FALLOUT SHELTER" sign. If no fallout shelter is available, go to a basement without windows or to the innermost room of a building. If you are at home, go to the basement or the innermost room on the lowest level to insulate yourself from the radioactivity as much as possible. Before entering any building, make sure the structure is not in imminent danger of collapsing.

Drought

Ways to Conserve Water

- Recycle your "used" water.
  - If the dog didn't drink all of his water, use it on houseplants.
  - Put a bucket in the shower to catch water from the showerhead; use it to hand-wash clothes.
  - Collect as much water as possible at every faucet instead of letting it go down the drain.
- Minimize dirty laundry to decrease the amount of water used by the washing machine.
- Limit the amount of electricity you use. Hydroelectric power plants obviously need lots of water to generate electricity, but coal-burning power plants and other types of power plants use water as well.

Bathroom

- Turn off the water while you brush your teeth or shave. Turn it on only when it's time to rinse.
- A bath in a tub uses the most water; a shower uses less water; a sponge bath uses the least.
- If you don't have a low-flush toilet, make yours into one by displacing some of the water in the tank. Place a rock or a plastic jug filled with gravel in the tank.

Kitchen

- Run the dishwasher only when it's full.
- If it takes a moment for very hot water or very cold water to reach the faucet, collect the water that comes out first and save it for drinking or cooking.
- A garbage disposal uses a lot of water. Instead of using it, make a compost pile for vegetable waste.

Laundry Room

- Run the clothes washer only when it's full. For small loads, adjust the water level to the size of the load.

Outdoors

♦ Sprinklers frequently waste a lot of water. If you use a sprinkler, start it in the early morning hours before dawn so the water can sink into the soil before the sun rises to dry it up. Watering at night is not recommended, as this encourages the development of plant diseases.

♦ Refrain from washing your car. If you have to wash your car, take it to a professional car wash where the water will be recycled.

♦ Be extremely careful with campfires, barbeques, fireworks, cigarettes, matches, etc.

♦ Collect rainwater in barrels (unless prohibited by local ordinances). Use it to water plants, wash cars, and fill the kids' pool.

Dust Storm/Sandstorm

On Foot

♦ Apply petroleum jelly to the insides of your nostrils to keep them from drying out.

♦ If you don't have a mask, wrap a bandana or other piece of cloth across your face. If you have plenty of water, moisten the cloth first.

♦ Take cover inside a building and wait out the storm. If no building is nearby, take shelter behind a rock, a tree, or anything else that can provide protection from the blasting force of the wind.

♦ Go to higher ground if you can find a safe spot where there is no danger from being struck by flying objects and if lightning isn't present. Don't go to lower ground or lie in a ditch, since flash flooding may occur, even if you don't see rain in your immediate area.

♦ Lie close to the ground and cover yourself with clothing or anything else that will offer protection from the windblown sand and flying objects.

♦ If you're in an area of dunes, stay on the windward side of the dunes to keep from being buried in sand (i.e., if the wind is coming from the west, stay on the western side of the dune).

In a Vehicle

♦ Pull to the side of the road or the safest place possible.

♦ Turn on your emergency flashers/hazard lights so other drivers can see you. Don't leave your taillights on, as other drivers may think you are moving and they might collide with you.

♦ Turn off the engine.

♦ Turn off heater or air conditioner.

♦ Close the windows and vents. Seal the vents with plastic and duct tape.

♦ Stay with your vehicle and wait until visibility improves so you can get back on the road.

Earthquake

Indoors

♦ If you are in a solid well-constructed building, get underneath a sturdy object, such as a desk or table, to protect yourself from falling objects.

♦ If you are in a flimsy poorly constructed building, lie in the fetal position next to a piece of furniture. If the walls and roof collapse around you, the furniture in the room may create a pocket of space that will protect you from being crushed.

♦ Stay away from windows, mirrors, or other objects that may shatter.

♦ Stay away from shelves, bookcases, entertainment centers, lockers, light fixtures, hanging pictures, or other large objects that could fall on you.

♦ Once the tremors stop, leave the building in case the structure has been damaged. Don't re-enter any building until it has been inspected and declared safe.

♦ Don't light matches or have other open flames in case of a natural gas leak.

Outdoors

♦ Avoid trees, power lines, underpasses, ramps, or other objects that could fall on you.

♦ Stay away from pipelines in case they are ruptured by the tremors.

♦ If you cannot seek shelter from falling objects, drop and cover. Crouch down and tuck yourself into a ball. Clasp your hands behind your neck and bury your face against your body. Close your eyes and cover your ears with your forearms.

♦ Don't enter any building until it has been inspected and declared safe.

In a Vehicle

♦ Stop your vehicle. Avoiding parking under trees, power lines, underpasses, ramps, or other objects that could fall on you. Stay away from pipelines in case they are ruptured by the tremors.

♦ If it's dark, turn on your emergency flashers/hazard lights so other drivers can see you. Don't leave your taillights on, as other drivers may think you are moving and they might collide with you.

♦ Stay in your vehicle and wait until the tremors stop.

♦ When the tremors stop, proceed with caution. Watch for buckled pavement, damaged bridges, and collapsing ramps.

Epidemic/Pandemic

♦ Avoid contact with the public as much as possible.

♦ If you must be out in public, wear a mask and gloves.

♦ Wash your hands thoroughly with soap and water when you return home from being out in public. Also wash your hands before handling food and before eating.

♦ Consider vaccination, if a vaccine is available.

Explosion/Airborne Release of an Unknown Substance

An explosion can result from a gas line break, a derailment of a train carrying hazardous chemicals, an accident at a chemical processing plant, a terrorist attack, or many other incidents. In all of these scenarios, you will have virtually no warning, so the best way to prepare is to remain aware of your surroundings and always know where the closest exit is.

An airborne release of some kind won't necessarily involve an explosion, but your response to the event should be similar to that for an explosion.

♦ If you are on public transportation or at a public venue, follow the instructions of crew members, facility supervisors, or emergency services personnel.

♦ If you have a respiratory mask, wear it. Otherwise, cover your nose and mouth with fabric, wet if possible. If you don't have fabric, use tissues or paper towels.

♦ Take shallow breaths and breathe in as little as possible until you are away from the disaster site.

♦ Open the windows if they are designed to open. If the windows do not open, don't waste your energy trying to break the glass, as modern glass is specially designed not to break easily.

♦ If you are on a plane and an oxygen mask drops from the ceiling, continuously press it tightly over your nose and mouth to achieve the best fit. If possible, seal the mask with a wet cloth. Breathe normally.

♦ If aboard ship, an open-air deck may be the safest place, as long as you can stay upwind of the release site.

♦ If debris is falling, protect yourself by crouching under a desk or table, or by covering yourself with a chair pad, empty drawer turned upside down, or whatever is available.

♦ Unless you are trying to open a window for fresh air or to escape, stay away from the windows. If you are outside, stay away from buildings with a large amount of glass. If a bomb has exploded, the windows may start raining glass down on you.

- Cover exposed skin.

- Try to keep your eyes closed as much as possible, unless it hinders your escape.

- Move as far as possible from the release site or the site of the breach in the structure.

- Leave the building, vehicle, or vessel as soon as possible. Do not pass through the spray or vapor if you can avoid it. If you must pass through it, hold your breath and move as quickly as possible. Once outside, go uphill and against or across the wind, if possible.

- If you are at work, report to your designated assembly point when you get out of the building.

- If you are trapped, do not shout, as that only makes you inhale dust. Instead:
  - Use a phone to call for help.
  - Tap on a wall or a pipe.
  - Flash a light to signal your location.

- Once you get away from the site of the incident, remove clothing and wash with soap and water as soon as possible.

- Listen to public broadcasts for updates on the situation. The federal government may release "push packs," a collection of drugs including antibiotics, antidotes, antitoxins, vaccines, and other medical supplies, stored strategically across the country so they can be delivered anywhere in the U.S. within 12 hours.

- Seek medical attention and decontamination if necessary.

- If you have been exposed to a chemical or radiological agent, the effects may be immediate or within a few hours or days.

- If you have been exposed to a biological agent, the effects may take days or even weeks to develop, so closely monitor any changes in health long-term.

Famine

Food may become scarce, or certain items may become so expensive that you can't afford them.

♦ Save money by cooking from scratch instead of buying prepared foods.

♦ Stock up on nonperishable items when they are on sale.

♦ Raise your own crops in a "crisis garden." If you don't have a plot of land, make it a container garden. Choose plants that are appropriate to your climate and nutrient-dense, and whatever produces the most food for the effort you put into it. Include ground plants, vines, fruit and nut trees, etc.

♦ Raise your own livestock. You may be able to raise fish, chickens, ducks, geese, turkeys, rabbits, bees, pygmy goats, and miniature cattle within city limits as long as you address restrictions regarding noise, smell, and sanitation. If you live outside the city limits, you can raise larger breeds as well as a larger variety of animals.

♦ Hunt, trap, and fish for food.

♦ Forage for berries, herbs, mushrooms, and other wild edibles.

These are the same skills you will need for your apocalypse plan. For more information on developing these skills, see the chapter entitled "Apocalypse Plan."

Financial Collapse

Every time you start to spend money, think about how you could achieve the same goal for less money.

- Decrease your expenses.
  - Cancel all nonessential services, such as cable or satellite TV, club memberships, magazine subscriptions, etc.
  - Eat food from home instead of from convenience stores and restaurants.
  - Buy food in bulk.
  - Buy generic products.
  - Reduce, reuse, and recycle. Reduce your consumption by using durable products rather than disposable. Reuse an item after it has served its original purpose, such as lining a trash can with a shopping bag. And finally, when an item can be used no more, recycle it by giving it to a waste processor who will convert it to another use.
  - Borrow movies and books from the library instead of paying to rent or buy them.
  - Buy used instead of new. Shop at thrift stores.
  - Ride your bicycle instead of using a motorized vehicle.
  - Carpool.
  - Have a staycation instead of a vacation.
  - Entertain at home instead of going out.
  - Visit museums, galleries, and zoos on their community outreach days when admission is free or a reduced price.
  - Have a picnic at a public park.
  - Give something of your own to someone you know will appreciate it, make your own gifts, or give the gift of your time.

- Increase your income with
  - part-time work
  - temporary work
  - contract work
  - freelance work

- Barter for goods and services.

- Clean out your closets, attic, basement, and garage. Have a yard sale, take your stuff to a consignment shop, or sell it online.

♦ Start your own business doing whatever you are capable of doing and meeting whatever needs your community has: babysitting, yard maintenance, bookkeeping, baking, catering, design, marketing, etc.

♦ Utilize community resources, if available.
  ♦ food banks
  ♦ subsidized housing
  ♦ subsidized utilities
  ♦ subsidized medical care

♦ Let your religious leader know about your situation and appeal to the members of your congregation for help.

Fire

If fire is approaching your home and you have time before escaping:

♦ Use a ladder to climb on the roof and wet down your house with a water hose.

♦ Spray fire-retardant gel or foam onto the exterior of your home.

Don't put your life at risk. Get away as soon as possible.

If you are surrounded by a wildfire and can't escape, do one of the following:

♦ Crouch in a body of water: a pond, a stream, or a drainage ditch.

♦ Cover yourself with wet clothing.

♦ Seek shelter in a cleared area with no combustible materials to feed the fire.

♦ Cover yourself with rocks and soil.

Flood

You're at risk from flooding if you occupy low-lying land near water, if you live downstream from a dam, if you live at the foot of a mountain with winter snowmelt, if you live in a climate with spring rains and summer thunderstorms, or if you live on a coast with the potential for tsunamis and hurricanes.

Flooding may be slow, giving you some time to prepare, such as when streams and rivers swell with snowmelt in the spring and gradually overflow their banks. Or flooding may be sudden, such as when a tsunami hits the coast or when a dam breaks.

◆ Stay alert to weather conditions. Listen to public broadcasts on TV or radio for advisories.

◆ Keep your distance from floodwaters.

◆ Go to higher ground.

◆ When you approach any bridge, check upstream before crossing. If the water volume is rising to the deck of the bridge, or the current is carrying large trees, rocks, or other debris, it's not safe to cross the bridge. Turn around and find another route.

◆ When in doubt about any flooding situation, remember this phrase: "Turn around, don't drown."

At Home or Work

◆ Use shovels to dig trenches to channel water away from the structure.

◆ If you evacuate:
  ◆ If you have time before you leave, turn off all gas lines. If floodwaters reach a gas appliance and extinguish the pilot flame but the gas continues to flow, your home or office would be at risk for an explosion and fire.
  ◆ If you have time before you leave, move files from bottom drawers to higher drawers or to shelves high off the floor.
  ◆ Take backup tapes, disks, CD's or flash drives of your computer files with you.
  ◆ Help the deaf, blind, and disabled.
  ◆ Go to higher ground.

On Foot

◆ Never try to walk through flooded areas. It takes only a few inches of moving water to knock you off your feet.

◆ If you fall into floodwaters, do not try to swim to safety, because the current will be too strong. Grab onto something stationary, such as a tree branch, or climb onto the roof of a house or car, and wait for help.

◆ Avoid contact with downed power lines.

◆ Watch for animals in the water, especially snakes. Mammals will be as panicked as you are, so don't approach them.

In a Vehicle

◆ Never try to drive through water. You cannot determine the condition of the road underneath the water, the depth of the water, or the speed of the current.

◆ If your vehicle stalls in water, immediately abandon it and get to higher ground. If you can't reach higher ground, open a window to let water in so the vehicle won't float, and then climb onto the roof and wait for help.

Hazardous Material Leak or Spill

A hazardous material leak or spill could result from a traffic accident involving a truck carrying hazardous materials, the derailment of a train carrying hazardous chemicals, an accident at a chemical processing plant, a terrorist attack, or some other incident. In all of these scenarios, you will have virtually no warning, so the best way to prepare is to remain aware of your surroundings, and always have an escape route in mind.

♦ If the leak or spill is outside of your building and you are advised to shelter-in-place, close off the building by shutting all exterior doors, windows, and vents. Seal with plastic and duct tape.

♦ If a leak or spill occurs inside your facility, put on an escape-pack respirator and leave immediately.

♦ If you are advised to evacuate out of the area, move upwind or crosswind of the leak or spill.

♦ Avoid ditches or other low places where vapor may collect.

Heat Wave

A heat wave occurs when the temperature is 10 degrees or more above normal for an extended period of time. Many combinations of climate and geography can experience a heat wave, but some areas are more vulnerable than others. Areas around a mountainside are susceptible, because air masses flowing down the slope can become compressed, increasing the temperature at the foot of the mountain. A heat wave can be more deadly in an urban area because of the concentration of dark pavement, closely crowded buildings that limit air circulation, lack of vegetation that would provide shade, and air pollution that traps hot air.

◆ Drink extra water.

◆ Drink an electrolyte or sports drink to replenish not only fluid but also essential minerals that are lost during perspiration.

◆ Since digestion raises your body temperature, eat smaller meals more frequently so your body will burn less energy all at once.

◆ Splash water on your face and body. When moisture on your skin evaporates, body heat goes with it.

◆ Wear lightweight, light-colored clothing.

◆ Cover exposed skin to protect it from the sun.

◆ Wear a wide-brimmed, vented hat. If you don't have a hat, wear a piece of cloth over your head and neck.

◆ Wear sunglasses. Sun reflecting off pavement, glass, or sand can produce a blinding glare.

◆ In the desert, before putting on your boots, check for creatures that may have crawled inside.

◆ In the desert, keep abrasive sand out of your boots by wrapping the tops of your boots with cloth.

◆ Plan your activities according to the rise and fall of the temperature. Refrain from strenuous work or exercise outdoors during the hottest part of the day. Stay in the shade, in front of a fan, or in air conditioning, if possible.

◆ Stay on the lowest floor of your building. Heat rises; the basement will be the coolest level.

◆ Close draperies, shades, and blinds on windows that receive morning or afternoon sun.

♦ If you don't have a fan or air conditioning, open your windows to allow air to circulate.

♦ If you don't have air conditioning, find out if your community has air-conditioned relief centers to go to. This is especially important for babies, the elderly, and people on certain kinds of medication.

♦ If official relief centers are not available, go to a public place that has air conditioning: a shopping mall, the library, the movies, a restaurant, etc.

♦ Go to the pool or a beach, but wear sunscreen, and shade yourself from the sun when you're not in the water.

♦ Do not leave children or pets in closed vehicles.

♦ Watch for signs of heat stroke.

Heat Stroke

Heat stroke is a life-threatening medical emergency. Seek medical attention immediately.

Symptoms:
♦ dry skin, lack of perspiration
♦ fast heart rate
♦ labored breathing
♦ dizziness and confusion
♦ convulsions
♦ unconsciousness

Treatment:
♦ Move to a cool area, in the shade.
♦ Remove clothing.
♦ Bathe in cool (not cold) water.
♦ Use a fan or air conditioner to aid in moisture evaporation.
♦ Drink water or an electrolyte beverage.
♦ Put on a cooling vest.

Hijacking or Other Hostage Situation

All terrorists on a mission may not reveal themselves at the same time. One may initially act alone to draw out security personnel or to find out who the "heroes" are among the hostages.

Your response to hostage-takers depends on their motives and demands.

If your captors are seeking ransom (money, weapons, an exchange for their imprisoned comrades, etc.), your goal is to stay alive until your release is negotiated or your captors are overcome.

♦ Remain composed. Be aware of what is happening around you and be prepared to act in case outsiders attempt to rescue you.
♦ Do not try to overcome your attackers.
♦ Do not try to escape unless you are positive you will be successful.
♦ Try to be inconspicuous. Avoid direct eye contact with your captors, and don't let them know you are watching them.
♦ Be passive and cooperative. Follow orders.
♦ If questioned, keep your answers short and to the point. Don't volunteer information that isn't asked.
♦ Be polite.
♦ Do not complain.
♦ Avoid unexpected movements.
♦ Remember: As long as you are alive and well, you are a valuable commodity to your captors.

If you are faced with suicide attackers who are determined to kill as many people as possible and inflict as much property damage as possible, it is imperative that you act quickly or you will die.

♦ If suspicious behavior appears to be escalating into a hostage-taking situation, shout for help to try to thwart the attack.
♦ Look among the other hostages for potential allies.
♦ Take the lead and quickly form the hostages into a group.
♦ Tell all of the hostages to throw whatever they have at the attackers' heads: handbags, briefcases, laptops, soda cans, books, magazines, backpacks, shoes, food trays, etc.
♦ Shield your body with whatever is available (seat cushions on a plane). Wrap clothing around your forearms for protection.
♦ Rush the attackers as a group; throw them down, and confine them.

Home Invasion

Perpetrators who break into homes are frequently looking for things they can sell to get the money to buy drugs. If a home invasion happens to you, you will be dealing with someone who is desperate, irrational, and possibly in a drug-altered state and out of touch with reality.

♦ Try to avoid a confrontation with the robber. Get out of the house by escaping through a door or window.

♦ If you can't get out, lock yourself in a room and call 911.

♦ If they have a gun, you have little choice but to cooperate. Encourage them to take whatever they want and leave.

♦ If they don't have a gun and they attack you personally, look for something you can use as a weapon. A weapon can be anything that gives you an advantage or places your adversary at a disadvantage.
  ♦ a fireplace tool or a log
  ♦ a vase, bowl, candlestick, or any object sitting on a table
  ♦ a lamp
  ♦ a potted plant
  ♦ kitty litter that you can throw in the eyes
  ♦ sports equipment, such as a golf club or a baseball bat

Hurricane

Evacuate if possible.

The greatest threat from a hurricane is not the wind but the water. Hurricane winds cause tides to rise higher than usual, creating a storm surge, the wall of water that causes deadly flooding.

If you plan to shelter-in-place:

♦ Install storm shutters on the windows.

♦ Outside, tie down loose objects or store them inside the garage or shed.

♦ Get inside your shelter. Close and brace all exterior doors.

♦ Fill tubs and sinks with water.

♦ Collect hand-cranked radio and flashlights. Avoid using candles or other open flames while the wind is blowing.

♦ Be prepared to start the generator and connect appliances you want to keep running.

♦ Close all interior doors.

♦ Get family and pets into the safe room. Bring valuables into your safe room: photographs, jewelry, and electronics.

♦ If you have to use an elevator or powered stair-lift to reach your safe room, get there as early as possible in case the power goes out, unless you have a battery backup.

♦ If you don't have a separate safe room, stay in an interior room. Put as many walls as possible between you and the exterior of the structure. Stay away from windows and glass doors.

♦ Notify your emergency contacts.

♦ Listen to the radio for updates.

♦ If your safe room is in the basement, keep an eye out for flooding. If water starts to rise, get out of the basement.

♦ Hurricanes move in a circular pattern. If the eye of the storm passes over you, you will get hit with high winds twice, once on the leading edge of the storm, and again on the trailing edge of the storm. Wait at least 30 minutes after the wind has passed before leaving your shelter.

♦ Watch for tornadoes, which can develop during or after a hurricane.

Landslides: Mudslides & Rockslides

Warning signs of an impending landslide:

- ♦ sounds of breaking tree limbs or tumbling rocks
- ♦ vibrations or rumbling of the earth
- ♦ bulging ground at the base of a slope
- ♦ water seeping to the surface
- ♦ new cracks in the sidewalk, driveway, pavement, or soil
- ♦ fences, walls, poles, or trees shifting from their normal position
- ♦ cracks appearing in the foundation, walls, or ceilings of structures
- ♦ doors and windows that start sticking

- ♦ If you're inside when a landslide occurs, stay inside. Move to the highest floor to try to stay above the debris, and take cover under a sturdy piece of furniture.
- ♦ If you're outside when a landslide occurs, run to higher ground away from the debris path.
- ♦ If you can't reach higher ground, take cover behind any object that might protect you, such as a tree.
- ♦ If you have no other way to protect yourself, curl into a ball and wrap your arms around your head.

Nuclear/Radiological Incident

Radiation may occur as the result of a leak, an explosion, an airborne release, or fallout. A "dirty bomb" uses common explosives to spread radioactive materials.

The effects of a nuclear explosion are:
♦ initial blast and pressure wave, which causes bone fractures and internal injuries or death
♦ thermal radiation, by direct absorption of heat, which causes flash burns, or by secondary fires in the environment, which cause flame burns
♦ nuclear radiation, which causes cell damage or death

Clues: Indications of a Possible Radiological Incident

♦ unusual metal debris, left from detonation of bomb
♦ material emitting heat without any sign of an external heating source
♦ material that is glowing
♦ dead animals, including mammals, birds, reptiles, insects, fish (manifestations may range from minutes to weeks)
♦ mass human casualties: unusually high number of individuals exhibiting similar unexplained symptoms, becoming sick or dying (manifestations may range from minutes to weeks)
♦ casualties that occur within a confined geographic area

If you are exposed to radiation, three factors are critical:

Time – Minimize the amount of time exposed to the radiation source.

Distance – Get as far away as possible from the source of the radiation.

Shielding – Create a barrier as thick as possible between you and the source of the radiation.

In the Event of a Nuclear Blast

♦ Do not look toward the site as it is happening. Shield your eyes to avoid temporary blindness or permanent eye damage.

♦ An electromagnetic pulse will disable all electrical and electronic devices in its path. Since any car, bus, train, or other vehicle with a computer chip will not start, your ability to escape quickly from the area will be greatly reduced. Be prepared to seek immediate shelter.

♦ Depending on the nature of the blast, you may have up to 15 minutes to get away from the blast zone before radioactive fallout starts raining down on you. Get as far away as possible from the detonation site, but find shelter before the fallout comes.

♦ Seek shelter underground. If you are in a public place, look for a yellow and black "FALLOUT SHELTER" sign. If no fallout shelter is available, go to a basement without windows or to the innermost room of a building. A concrete and/or brick building offers more protection than one made of wood or metal. If you are at home, go to the basement or the innermost room on the lowest level to insulate yourself from the radioactivity as much as possible. Before entering any building, make sure the structure is not in imminent danger of collapsing.

♦ Once you reach shelter, remove your clothes and seal them in plastic bags. If possible, remove clothes outside; do not take them into your shelter.

♦ Wash with soap and water, but do not scrub the skin. Do not use conditioner in your hair, as this makes it more difficult to rinse out radioactive particles.

♦ Take potassium iodide if instructed to do so.

At Home

- Remove contaminated clothing and get inside with children and pets.
- Wash off with soap and water.
- Close and lock all outside doors, windows and vents.
- Go to the basement or the innermost room on the lowest level to insulate yourself from the radioactivity as much as possible.
- Listen to the radio or TV or access the Internet for updates on what areas have been exposed, what symptoms to watch for, and what to do if you think you have been exposed.
- Stay inside until the level of radioactivity has dropped.
- If you become sick, seek medical attention as soon as possible.
- Be prepared to evacuate.

In a Vehicle

- As long as the engine is running:
  - Head away from the disaster site as quickly as possible; head upwind or crosswind.
  - Turn off heater or air conditioner.
  - Close the windows and vents.
  - Listen to the radio for updates from the authorities.

- If your vehicle becomes disabled, get out and seek shelter underground.
  - If you are in a public place, look for a black and yellow "FALLOUT SHELTER" sign.
  - If no fallout shelter is available, go to a basement without windows or to the innermost room of a building.
  - Before entering any building, make sure the structure is not in imminent danger of collapsing.
  - If no buildings are available, lie flat on the ground until the shock wave passes. Then seek shelter.

In Public

♦ Depending on the nature of the blast, you may have up to 15 minutes to get away from the blast zone before radioactive fallout starts raining down on you. Get as far away as possible from the detonation site, but find shelter before the fallout comes.

♦ Travel in a direction that will lead you away from the site of the disaster, against the wind and uphill, if possible.

♦ Travel on foot. All vehicular transportation will become disabled.

♦ Seek shelter underground. Look for a yellow and black "FALLOUT SHELTER" sign. If no fallout shelter is available, go to a basement without windows or to the innermost room of a building. Before entering any building, make sure the structure is not in imminent danger of collapsing.

♦ Once you reach shelter, remove your clothes and seal them in plastic bags. If possible, remove clothes outside; do not take them into your shelter.

♦ Wash off with soap and water.

♦ Listen to the TV or radio for updated information from authorities. Follow their instructions on medical treatment and environmental decontamination.

♦ Stay inside until the level of radioactivity has dropped.

♦ If you become sick, seek medical attention as soon as possible.

♦ Be prepared to evacuate.

♦ Help the deaf, blind, and disabled.

Children

◆ Closely monitor children who have been exposed to radiation. Since they are still growing, their cells are dividing rapidly, and radiation can disrupt the growth process.

◆ Children are more likely than adults to become dehydrated from vomiting and diarrhea. If they experience these symptoms, be sure they receive plenty of fluids.

Pets

◆ Like people, pets should not go outside during radiological emergencies.

◆ If pets may be contaminated, they should be washed thoroughly with soap and water before bringing them inside your shelter.

◆ If you are evacuating, your pets will be safest evacuating, too. You have no guarantee of when, if ever, you will be able to return home.

Shooting

A shooting may be the result of terrorism, workplace violence, or criminal activity such as a robbery.

♦ If you hear gunshots or see an attack start to unfold, get away if at all possible. Don't try to reason with the perpetrator.

♦ If you can't get away, hide.
  ♦ If you are indoors, lock the door of the room you are in, and stay away from the door and windows. Hide in a closet, under a desk, or behind any barrier available.
  ♦ If you are outdoors, take cover behind or underneath a solid object.

♦ Get down and stay down. Drop to the floor or ground, and stay as low as possible.

♦ Remain still until you are certain the danger has passed. Be as obscure and quiet as you possibly can. Don't do anything to draw attention to yourself.

♦ If you must change locations, crawl on your stomach.

Thunderstorm

♦ If you can hear thunder, the storm is close enough to put you in danger.

♦ Put pets and livestock inside a building.

♦ Take cover immediately inside a building or a vehicle.

♦ If you are caught outside and cannot reach a building or vehicle:
  ♦ Do not stand under a tree.
  ♦ Do not stand out in the open.
  ♦ Do not lie flat on the ground.
  ♦ Crouch down and hold your knees against your chest to make yourself into a small ball. Minimize your contact with the ground as much as possible. Do not touch the ground with your hands.

♦ Avoid contact with sinks, showers, or tubs during a thunderstorm.

♦ Avoid contact with electrical equipment or phones.

Besides the electrical danger, hail may occur during a thunderstorm. Getting hit with hail falling from the sky at a high velocity can be deadly. Get inside if possible.

Tornado

Watch for signs that a tornado is about to touch down:
- a roaring sound, like a freight train
- dead calm
- swirling debris
- greenish cast to the sky

Tornadoes develop quickly. You will most likely have only enough time to seek shelter and time for little else.

The safest place in any building is, in descending order:

1. fireproof and waterproof safe room
2. basement, cellar, or other underground structure
3. windowless interior room such as a hall, closet, or bathroom on the ground floor

In Public

- If you are caught in a multi-story building when a tornado strikes, go to the lowest floor available. First choice: basement. Second choice: ground floor
- Avoid taking shelter in large buildings with wide roof spans that could easily collapse, such as shopping malls, supermarkets, or "big-box" stores.
- Do not use elevators in case the power goes out.

On Foot

- Lie flat in a ditch or other low area. However, ditches and other low spots are susceptible to flooding from the rainstorms that accompany tornadoes. Beware of areas that can become drowning hazards.

In Your Vehicle

- Get out and seek shelter. Do not stay in your vehicle, since it can be tossed around by the wind in a tornado.
- If no shelter is available, lie flat on the ground.

At Home

- Get inside your shelter. If you live in a mobile home, get out and find safer shelter.
- Close and brace all exterior doors.
- Do not open windows in your house, as this is likely to cause more damage, not less.
- Close all interior doors.
- If you have time, collect hand-cranked radio and flashlights. Avoid using candles or other open flames while the wind is blowing.
- If you have time, notify your emergency contacts.
- Get family and pets into the safe room.
- If you have to use an elevator or powered stair-lift to reach your safe room, get there as early as possible in case the power goes out.
- If you don't have a separate safe room, stay in an interior room. Put as many walls as possible between you and the exterior of the structure. Stay away from windows and glass doors.
- Get underneath a sturdy object, such as a desk or table, to protect yourself from flying debris.
- If you have no other protection, sit facing a wall with your knees tucked into your chest and your head down. Clasp your hands behind your neck and bury your face against your body. Close your eyes and cover your ears with your forearms.
- Avoid corners because they trap debris.
- If your safe room is in the basement, keep an eye out for flooding. If water starts to rise, get out of the basement.
- Listen for updates on your NOAA radio and remain in your shelter until you are absolutely sure that the danger has passed. Tornadoes can backtrack or change direction in seconds.

Tsunami

A tsunami consists of a series of large waves traveling with great force. They are caused by underwater earthquakes, volcanoes, or other disturbances. You are at greatest risk next to a coast that is along fault lines where earthquakes are likely to occur.

♦ If you notice a rapid rise or fall of coastal waters, move inland and seek higher ground.

♦ Tsunamis produce multiple waves. Stay away from the beach and listen to your NOAA radio to find out when the danger has passed.

♦ If you are trapped by floodwaters, do not try to swim to safety, because the current will be too strong. Grab onto something stationary, such as a tree branch, or climb onto the roof of a house or car, and wait for help.

Volcano

Volcanoes can erupt with very little warning, but scientists keep an eye on them by measuring nearby earthquake activity, gas emissions, and ground deformation. Volcanoes can produce slow-moving lava or erupt in a violent, catastrophic explosion. Volcanoes are classified by stages:

normal – a volcano in a non-eruptive state

advisory – a volcano showing elevated unrest

watch – a volcano with escalating unrest with increased potential for eruption, or a minor eruption already underway that poses limited hazards

warning – a highly hazardous eruption is imminent or already underway

The dangers from a volcanic eruption include
- lava flow
- ash
- poisonous gases
- hurtling rocks that kill by impact, burial, or heat
- climate change (volcanic winter) that results in crop failure and death of livestock, leading to famine and possibly mass extinctions, depending on its severity

The most dangerous area is the 20-mile radius around a volcano. The danger zone may extend to 100 miles or more, depending on the wind.

- If you are in the path of a lava flow, or close enough to a spewing volcano to be affected by heavy ash, poisonous gases, or flying debris, evacuate immediately.

- Don't drive through ash, since it can clog the engine and cause your vehicle to stall.

- Store vehicles and machinery in a garage or shed to avoid damage from ash.

Even if you don't have to evacuate, you may be affected by wind-blown ash.

♦ Put pets inside the house or garage and livestock inside a barn to protect them from ash.

♦ Get inside with children.

♦ Close exterior doors, windows, and vents.

♦ Unpack your plastic sheeting to cover the openings of your shelter. Using duct tape, secure each plastic sheet at the corners, and then seal the edges. Cover all doors, windows, and vents. At the bottom edges of doors, extend the plastic a few inches into the room at a right angle over the floor to make sure the gap between the door and the threshold is sealed off.

♦ If you don't have plastic sheeting, close the draperies, curtains, blinds, or shades.

♦ Listen to the radio or TV or access the Internet for updates on what areas are being affected and to monitor changes in wind direction.

♦ If ash collects on the roof of your dwelling, sweep it off to avoid the roof's collapsing.

♦ If you have to go outside, wear protective clothing. Wear long pants, long sleeves, and gloves. Wear a mask, or cover your nose and mouth with a damp cloth. Wear goggles to protect your eyes, and earplugs or earmuffs to protect your ears.

Vog (a contraction of "volcanic smog") is a cloud of fumes consisting of rather unpleasant sulfuric acid aerosols. If vog is present, stay inside with windows and doors sealed. Use an air conditioner or dehumidifier to condense water and sulfur compounds out of the air. Or saturate a piece of cloth with a paste of baking soda and water and drape it over a fan at low speed to neutralize the sulfur compounds. **CAUTION:** When using electrical appliances near water, be careful not to get the motor wet.

Water Emergency: capsized/sinking boat or plane crash

Abandoning the Disabled Craft

◆ Abandon the disabled craft as soon as possible. Use the time before it sinks to gather supplies and launch a life raft.

◆ Keep your clothes on.

◆ Before you go overboard, grab a flotation device (life jacket, life ring, seat cushion, etc.). If you don't have a manufactured flotation device, make one from clothing. Fill shirtsleeves or pant legs with air and tie off the openings of the garment to make an air sac.

◆ Take an emergency kit with you. If you don't have an emergency kit, take warm clothing and fruit, snacks, or other portable food.

◆ Once you are in the water, try to climb into a life raft or lifeboat. If none is available, look for floating debris that you can use for flotation.

◆ Swim or paddle upwind away from the listing craft. As it sinks, a large object such as a boat or plane will suck nearby objects, including you, under the surface of the water.

◆ If oil is burning on the water's surface, swim or paddle around it. If you are in the water and you can't swim around it, swim under it. Deflate your life jacket to go underwater. If you need to come up for air before you clear the patch of burning oil, push the water aside from beneath the surface to create an opening.

Launching a Life Raft or Life Boat

Depending on the emergency provisions, you may have access to an inflated open raft, a deflated covered raft that comes in a canister, or a rigid dinghy.

◆ Follow crew instructions to launch a rigid dinghy that employs a mechanical system.

◆ Before launching the raft or boat, tie your bags containing emergency supplies to it so they won't be lost if they fall overboard. Once you are in the raft or boat, you will be able to pull in the line to retrieve your bags and bring them onboard.

◆ If you are launching a raft, tie it to the craft you are abandoning so the raft doesn't float or blow away. For a raft that comes in a canister, you can use the rip cord for this purpose.

- Throw the raft into the water downwind so it won't be blown into the craft you are abandoning. A raft that comes in a canister is equipped with a long rip chord so it can float a safe distance away from a disabled craft.

- A raft that comes in a canister inflates automatically using bottled carbon dioxide. If the raft doesn't inflate automatically, use the backup hand pump.

- Extra carbon dioxide escapes through over-pressure valves in the tubes of the raft. The raft is equipped with screw-in plugs to stop gas leaks if these valves leak.

- If the raft doesn't maintain pressure, find the leak and fix it using the repair kit that comes with the raft.

- Ensure that the floor of the raft is inflated to insulate you from the cold water. It also allows the raft to self-bail. This means that water splashing over the sides into the raft will be drained out.

- If you can't get directly into the raft, jump into the water. Grab the handles on the raft to pull yourself in, or tip the raft up on one end, put one knee inside the raft, lean in, and let the raft fall back to the surface of the water.

- If the raft is upside down in the water, attach a line to the side of the raft, move to the side opposite of where it is attached, and pull it over to be right side up.

- If you need more maneuverability, tie your life vest to your body or to the raft and then remove it until you get into the raft.

- On covered rafts, the canopy has a pocket with a knife that you can use to cut the rip cord that you used to tie the raft to the disabled craft.

- Wait until you are a safe distance from the disabled craft to deploy a sea anchor or drogue.

Conserving Body Heat

If you are floating in the water, you must try to conserve body heat to avoid hypothermia. Roll yourself into a ball by crossing your legs at the ankles and drawing your legs up against your body, keeping only your head above water.

Survival at Sea

Life rafts may be equipped with water, food, a fishing kit, first aid supplies, a raft repair kit, a flashlight with spare batteries and a spare bulb, a signal mirror, signaling flares, a radio beacon, and other survival gear. In a life raft, your priorities are to:
  ♦ protect yourself from the elements
  ♦ find drinking water
  ♦ make yourself visible so you can be rescued
  ♦ reach land if possible

♦ If you are cold:
  ♦ close the sea curtains on the side of the prevailing wind
  ♦ remove wet clothing and allow it to dry

♦ If you are hot:
  ♦ open the sea curtains on the side of the prevailing wind
  ♦ stay out of direct sunlight; wear thin clothing to protect against sunburn
  ♦ during the day, dampen your clothes to help stay cool

♦ Salvage useful items floating in the water and tie them to the raft.

♦ Tie one person to the raft to keep it from blowing away in case it capsizes.

♦ In heavy weather, throw the drogue off the stern of the boat to keep it from capsizing. Use a piece of rope that is half the length of the prevailing waves, so that the drogue goes down a wave as the boat goes up a wave.

♦ Divide tasks, such as fishing, distilling water, navigating, signaling, etc.

♦ Paddle toward other rafts and tie them together for higher visibility.

Water

♦ If your water supplies are low, don't drink water for the first 24 hours.

♦ Catch rain in any available container.

♦ Use desalination supplies if available in the raft.

♦ Use a solar still if one is available.

♦ Minimize physical exertion, especially during the hottest parts of the day, to retain as much water in your body as possible.

♦ If you feel nauseous, take motion sickness medication. Vomiting causes a heavy loss of water from the body.

♦ Don't drink alcohol, as it will dehydrate you.

♦ Water from sea ice is saltier than freshwater, but sea ice can be consumed on a short-term basis without damage to most humans. Water from an iceberg is freshwater, but approaching an iceberg is extremely dangerous.

♦ Don't drink saltwater. The salt content is too high. It will kill you.

Food

♦ Eat food only if you have sufficient drinking water. Your body requires water to process food, so the less you eat, the less water you require. Most healthy people can survive many days without food.

♦ Ration whatever food you have.

♦ Eat seaweed only if it is firm to the touch. Do not eat seaweed that appears to be rotting.

♦ You can fish with a hooked line, a net, or a spear. If you don't have a spear, make one by binding a knife to an oar or pole.

♦ Wear gloves or cover your hands with a shirt to protect against cuts when handling sharp objects such as a hook, knife, scales, or spines.

♦ Protect the raft from sharp objects such as fishing hooks or spears.

♦ Use a net to catch small fish, either to eat or to use as bait for larger fish.

♦ Be careful not to capsize the boat while catching large fish.

♦ A large school of fish provides easy fishing, but it also attracts predators such as sharks and barracuda. Don't fish if predators are nearby.

♦ Gut the fish as soon as you catch it to protect the quality of the meat.

♦ If you aren't going to eat the fish immediately, sun-dry it for later.

Predators

♦ If you are in a raft, avoid dangling your arms and legs over the side.

♦ If you are bleeding, treat the wound to stop the flow of blood. Do not allow blood to trickle into the water.

♦ If you feel nauseous, take motion sickness medication. If you vomit, collect it in the raft and then throw it overboard as far behind the raft as possible.

♦ Limit the amount of urine and feces that gets dumped into the water in one place. Do not leave a trail of human waste for predators to follow.

♦ If approached by a predator, try to drive it away by slapping the water, shouting, or hitting it with an object. If you are in the water with other people, form a ring facing outward and make noise.

Rescue

Try to reach land or to be seen on the water.

♦ If you are within sight of land, swim or paddle toward shore. If you are in the water, rest by floating on your back.

♦ If you are in a remote area, your best chance of rescue is to remain close to the area where radio contact was last made before disaster struck. Throw a sea anchor off the bow of the boat to remain in the area of the wreckage for at least 72 hours.

♦ Have signaling equipment such as mirrors or flares ready to use. Use them only when search planes or ships are within range.

Making Headway/Covering Distance

Rigid dinghies may have a motor. An inflatable raft may have a sail.
Without a motor or sail, you will have to rely on currents. The raft will be
moved by a combination of wind current and water current.
- Wind current has more effect on a raft that sits high in the water.
- Water current has more effect on a raft that sits low in the water.

Assess the wind and water conditions and act accordingly.

- If the wind is heavy, the wind current is probably going to help you
  cover a greater distance than the water current. To take advantage of
  the wind current, make the raft as light as possible by throwing any
  unnecessary items overboard.

- If the wind is light, the water current is probably going to help you cover
  a greater distance than the wind current. To take advantage of the
  water current, keep as much weight in the raft as possible.

Navigation

If you know approximately where you are, you will have some idea of which
direction to head to find help. If you don't have a compass or sextant, you
can navigate using one of the following methods:

Watch

In the northern latitudes, the sun passes across the sky south of you. If you
are in the northern hemisphere, aim the hour hand of a watch at the sun.
The point that is halfway between twelve o'clock and the hour hand is the
direction of south.

In the southern latitudes, the sun passes across the sky north of you. If you
are in the southern hemisphere, aim twelve o'clock on a watch at the sun.
The point that is halfway between twelve o'clock and the hour hand is the
direction of north.

The watch must be running accurately on local time. The most reliable
results occur at noon every day. This method is most reliable between 40°-
60° north or south of the equator. The closer you are to the equator, the
less reliable this method becomes.

Sun

The sun rises in the east and sets in the west. At the equator, it rises due east and sets due west. At higher latitudes, it will be slightly off of due east or due west, but generally speaking, if the rising sun is on your right, then east is to your right, north is in front of you, west is to your left, and south is behind you.

Stars

Polaris, the North Star, appears in the sky over the North Pole and is used for navigation in the northern hemisphere. The North Star is at the tip of the handle of the Little Dipper, which is located opposite the Big Dipper. Draw an imaginary line from the North Star to the earth below it, and you have located the direction of north.

The Southern Cross (four stars that represent the points of a cross) is used for navigation in the southern hemisphere. It is located near two bright stars called the Pointers. Draw an imaginary line from the top of the cross to the bottom; then extend this line from the bottom by a length that is 4 ½ times the distance between those two stars. From that point, draw an imaginary line to the earth below it, and you have located the direction of south.

Sighting Land

♦   Watch birds. They generally fly away from land in the morning and toward land in the afternoon and evening.

♦   Look for floating vegetation or debris that would indicate the presence of land and civilization nearby.

♦   Look for clouds in an otherwise cloudless sky. This may indicate the existence of a land mass, as heat from the ground can lead to cloud formation.

♦   Look for greenish clouds that may be reflecting lagoon water. A lagoon would indicate the existence of land.

During Disaster

Landing

If you believe the land is inhabited, signal for rescue and wait for help to come to you.

If you want to make landfall on your own:

- Approach from the leeward side of an island (the opposite side from which the wind is blowing, i.e., if the wind is blowing from the west, approach the island from the east).
- Stay clear of rocks and heavy surf.
- Ride the crests of waves until you reach the beach; remain in the raft until it is grounded.
- If you are carried back out to sea by a rip tide, don't try to swim or paddle directly against it; wait until it dissipates and try again to reach the shore.
- If coming in over coral reefs, wear shoes to avoid cutting your feet when you get out of the raft.

Communications

If you don't have any telecommunications equipment, you will have to make contact with rescuers with a visual signal or one that is audible from a distance.

- Set off flares if they are within range of being seen.
- Build a fire and create smoke.
- Lay out rocks or logs in a large formation: X or SOS
- Signal SOS with a mirror or flashlight or with a horn.
- Display signals in groups of three: three piles of rocks or three fires.
- Display signal flags "N" and "C" together to indicate distress.
- Display a square flag with a ball or other circular object.
- Create an unusual visual display to attract attention.
- If a vehicle, aircraft, or watercraft is in sight, raise both arms at an angle to indicate "Y," as in "Yes, I need help," or wave both arms above your head.

Winter Storms – Snow, Ice, Cold

At Home

♦ If you shovel snow, take frequent breaks to avoid overexertion.
♦ Cover your mouth with a scarf or ski mask to warm the air you breathe into your lungs.
♦ Cover all exposed skin.
♦ If your clothes get wet, change into dry clothes to retain body heat.
♦ Never use a blowtorch or other open-flame device to thaw pipes.
♦ Never fill a kerosene heater inside. Let the heater cool and take it outside to refill it.
♦ Keep space heaters away from draperies, furniture, and other flammable objects.

On Foot

♦ Cover your mouth with a scarf or ski mask to warm the air you breathe into your lungs.
♦ Cover all exposed skin.
♦ Seek shelter as soon as possible.

In Your Vehicle

If you are stranded, make your vehicle visible to rescuers.

♦ Turn your headlights on, but only while running the engine so you don't run the battery down.
♦ Tie the emergency banner from your emergency kit to the antenna; if you don't have a banner, any piece of brightly colored fabric will work.
♦ Once the snow has stopped falling, open the hood of your vehicle to signal to passersby that you need help.

Workplace Violence

Workplace violence may be committed by criminals who have no relationship to the organization (for example, an armed robber who steals cash or drugs), disgruntled customers who are dissatisfied with a product or service, employees who are frustrated with the organization's policies or other workers, especially supervisors, or individuals who have a personal relationship with one of the organization's employees.

Occupations and workplaces with a high risk of violence are:
♦ police officers
♦ correctional officers
♦ social service workers
♦ health care workers
♦ public workers, especially inspectors and code enforcement officials
♦ organizations with a high number of minimum-wage workers
♦ organizations with poor working conditions and lack of job security
♦ organizations that tolerate sexual harassment and discrimination

If you or a co-worker is threatened, report it to someone high enough in management to do something about it. Also report it to the police.

If violence erupts without warning:

♦ If you hear gunshots or see an attack start to unfold, get away if at all possible. Don't try to reason with the perpetrator, regardless of how well you know the person.
♦ If you can't get away, hide.
  ♦ If you are indoors, lock the door of the room you are in, and stay away from the door and windows. Hide in a closet, under a desk, or behind any barrier available.
  ♦ If you are outdoors, take cover behind or underneath a solid object.
♦ Get down and stay down. Drop to the floor or ground, and stay as low as possible.
♦ Remain still until you are certain the danger has passed. Be as obscure and quiet as you possibly can. Don't do anything to draw attention to yourself.
♦ If you must relocate, crawl on your stomach.
♦ Call 911 if you can do so without attracting the attention of the perpetrator.

Section 3

After Disaster

This section outlines what to do after the acute phase of the disaster has passed.

If you will be able to re-establish a "normal" life, Chapter 11 helps you implement the recovery plan that you developed.

If an apocalyptic event forever changes your lifestyle and the world around you, Chapter 12 helps you implement the apocalypse plan that you developed.

Chapter 11

Recovery

Exactly when does "after" begin? It depends on how the crisis plays out. The beginning of "after" may be clear-cut, or it may be imprecise.

If a fire destroys your home, the "end" of the event happens when the fire trucks pull away. The recovery period begins at that moment.

When the tremors stop after an earthquake, you may consider that to be the "end" of the event and start cleaning up. But aftershocks can last for days, and you may have to start over. Recovery may begin more than once.

If the power grid fails or is attacked, you and others could be without power for weeks or months. We immediately think of being without light and either heat or air conditioning, but our lives are heavily dependent on electricity to operate our phones, computers, TV's, radios, refrigeration, water pumps, sewage-treatment facilities, gas pumps, cash registers, ATM's, traffic lights, rail systems, air service, and more. In such a scenario, you may need to make temporary adjustments to the way you live and learn to do things a different way until power is restored. Recovery may begin in stages.

What does "recovery" mean?

If damages can be repaired and you can return to the life you had before the catastrophe, the aftermath of the disaster may be relatively easy to deal with. You may have to clean up some things yourself, or you may need to file an insurance claim and deal with contractors to repair damages, or you may need to apply for federal disaster aid. Although it may involve a lot of time, money, and hard work, ultimately you'll be able to live in the same place and work at the same job, and life will return to "normal."

On the other hand, if the disaster results in life-altering changes, the aftermath will be more difficult to deal with, in terms of the practical aspects of daily living, financial hardship, and emotional stress. If your property is washed away in a mudslide and you have no lot left to rebuild on, you will be forced to relocate, without any of your belongings. Or in the event of radioactive contamination, your home may be intact but uninhabitable. You would be forced to relocate, without any of your belongings. You may have to move far away from family and friends and may have to change jobs. In these scenarios, you will have to adjust to a "new normal."

GENERAL

♦ Listen to radio or TV broadcasts for continuing updates.

♦ If you become injured or sick, seek medical treatment as soon as possible.

♦ After a major disaster, local repair contractors will be overwhelmed, so be patient. Beware of hiring contractors from out of the area; they may take your deposit and disappear. Even if you hire a legitimate contractor from out of the area, the work may not pass inspection if the contractor isn't familiar with your local building codes. Your choices are to wait for a reputable contractor in your area, or start doing some of the work yourself. Inspectors will also be overwhelmed. If you need a permit to proceed, you will have no choice but to wait for them.

♦ Make your own all-purpose cleaner using **EITHER** chlorine bleach **OR** ammonia mixed with water. The higher the concentration of the chemical, the more powerful it will be. Keep the area well ventilated to lessen the concentration of fumes.

☠ **WARNING: NEVER MIX CHLORINE AND AMMONIA TOGETHER, BECAUSE THIS PRODUCES DEADLY FUMES.**

ANIMALS

♦ Avoid animals that have been displaced by the disaster. They may be sick or injured and they may bite. If you need to have an animal removed from your property, contact local animal control authorities.

♦ If an animal bites you, get medical attention immediately. Also contact animal control authorities so the animal can be quarantined.

♦ If animal carcasses remain on your property after the disaster, wear gloves to bury them or contact local authorities for assistance in the disposal of dead animals.

PUBLIC AREAS

♦ Avoid downed power lines.

♦ Stay away from gas lines in case they are ruptured. Do not have an open flame if a gas leak may be present.

♦ Avoid broken water lines. Floodwaters may carry disease, chemicals, and raw sewage. The water may also be electrically charged from downed power lines, even if you can't see them.

♦ Do not try to wade or swim through moving water. The current is strong and it will overcome you.

♦ If you come in contact with floodwaters, wash with soap and water as soon as possible.

♦ Beware of areas where floodwaters have receded. Roads and bridges may have weakened and may collapse under the weight of a car.

HOME OR WORK

- Check for structural damage before reentering your home. Check the foundation, walls, and ceilings for cracks. If your home has been hit by an intense event such as a fire, tornado, hurricane, or flooding, hire a professional to do the inspection. When you go in:

  - Wear a hardhat, mask, safety glasses, gloves, long sleeves and long pants, and sturdy, waterproof boots.

  - Beware of broken glass and protruding objects.

  - Beware of slippery floors and steps.

  - If your home is flooded, watch for snakes and alligators as well as other displaced marine life and land animals.

- If you see exposed wires, call a professional electrician.

- If you have gas lines on your property, do not have any open flames until you have determined if any leaks are present. If you smell gas or hear hissing, leave immediately and call the gas company.

- If you see broken pipes, call a professional plumber.

- Even if your water pipes appear to be intact, purify your water until you have confirmed that your water supply is not contaminated.

- If you have been without power for more than 24 hours, use the food in your refrigerator immediately or discard it. If you have been without power for more than 48 hours, use the food in your freezer immediately or discard it.

- Check for spillage of chemicals stored on your property.

    - If a spill is minor, you may clean it up yourself.

        * Wear protective gear (mask, safety glasses, rubber gloves, rubber boots).

        * Put barriers around floor drains to protect them.

        * Absorb the spill using absorbents appropriate to the material (oil absorbent pads, granular clay, kitty litter).

        * Seal contaminated material in a plastic bag and tag it with the contents.

        * Take contaminated materials to a hazardous waste treatment facility.

    - If any of the following apply, call your local Environmental Protection Agency:

        * you don't know what the spilled material is

        * the material is toxic or flammable

        * the spill is too large to contain

        * you don't have the necessary protective gear (mask, safety glasses, gloves, boots)

        * you don't have the equipment necessary to do the job safely

- Take photos of damage and file claims with your insurance company for your home and contents, vehicles, or other personal property. You may have to wait for an adjustor before beginning cleanup and repairs. Follow the instructions of your insurance company so you don't forfeit any benefits.

- Replant damaged ground as soon as possible to reduce erosion and further damage.

- Seek assistance from relief organizations. Governmental agencies and private charities will issue public announcements about how and where to seek aid.

AFTER A FLOOD

♦ Open doors and windows to increase ventilation.

♦ Set fans in doorways and windows to blow outward.

♦ Use a dehumidifier to remove excess moisture from the air.

♦ Use a wet-vac or pump to draw up standing water.

♦ Discard curtains, area rugs, upholstered furniture, mattresses, and pillows. If you want to try to save these items, dry them in the sun and spray with disinfectant, or have them professionally cleaned.

♦ Wash or dry-clean all clothing, towels, and bedding.

♦ Remove and discard wall-to-wall carpeting and padding.

♦ Wash and disinfect hard, non-porous surfaces made of concrete, stone, brick, glass, or plastic, such as floors, walls, countertops, and bathroom tile. Wash with soap and water, and then rinse with a mixture of chlorine and water OR ammonia and water. A 10% solution is recommended to kill most bacteria and viruses. Mix 1 part chemical with 9 parts water. ☠ **WARNING:** Do not mix chlorine and ammonia together.

♦ Building materials that have absorbed water must be replaced. This includes paneling, drywall, and insulation. Remove wallboard at least one foot above the visible water line left by the flood. Air out the interior spaces between walls completely before replacing the wallboard.

♦ Have your heating/ventilation/air conditioning system cleaned by a professional.

♦ Have your septic system serviced by a professional.

♦ Discard contaminated articles that cannot be disinfected. Seal them in plastic bags to prevent the spread of mold.

♦ Don't eat food that has come in contact with floodwater.

AFTER AN EARTHQUAKE

◆ If you live in a coastal area, stay away from the beach and be on the lookout for tsunamis.

◆ Be careful opening cabinets and closets. Items may fall out on top of you.

◆ Have the chimney inspected before lighting a fire.

AFTER A FIRE

◆ Open your safe only after it has cooled. Opening a hot safe can be dangerous.

◆ Check for remaining embers or sparks that could reignite the fire.

Chapter 12

Apocalypse

The nature of the disaster and the amount of destruction it causes will determine how to respond. In the face of cataclysmic change, you must be prepared to evacuate, to relocate permanently, to produce your own food, to build your own shelter, and to make your own clothing. You must be prepared to do whatever it takes to care for yourself and your family.

In some post-apocalyptic situations, you may be able to stay in your home, but you may be forced to make substantial changes to the way you live. For instance, a widespread and long-term shutdown of the power grid could occur. In this case, your shelter would be intact, but the delivery systems for water, food, and other goods and services would be radically altered.

In other post-apocalyptic situations, you may be forced to relocate to a different geographic area. For instance, radiological contamination could make your home uninhabitable for decades. Or the eruption of a super-volcano could bring on a widespread volcanic winter. In these cases, you may be sharing a relatively small land area overcrowded with too many survivors to support, leading to fierce competition for scarce resources.

Whatever the situation, you may need to build or rebuild some or all of the following facilities and systems to meet your basic survival needs:

- ◆ shelter
- ◆ water
- ◆ food
- ◆ clothing
- ◆ energy
- ◆ waste disposal
- ◆ security

Explaining in detail how to build and maintain such structures is beyond the scope of this little book, but the following pages give you an overview. Consult your library of reference books to help you construct the accommodations and learn the techniques you need to survive.

SHELTER

If you are on the move, you will need temporary shelter as you travel. Even after you reach your destination, you may need temporary shelter while you look for or build a permanent shelter.

A temporary shelter can be a tent or bivouac sack that you carry with you, or something that you make out of materials available in your environment. Likewise, your permanent shelter will have to be constructed of whatever is available, such as:

- animal hides
- dried animal dung
- tall grasses or other plant stalks
- leaves and branches
- logs
- plywood
- sod
- rammed earth
- dried mud
- fired brick
- stone
- concrete
- glass
- plastic
- foam
- corrugated sheet metal
- abandoned bus or train car
- abandoned building
- shipping container

PERMANENT WATER TREATMENT

Whether you are on the move or settled down, you will have to assume that all surface water is contaminated until you have had a chance to treat it. Water that looks and smells clean may, in fact, be contaminated, and water that looks and smells dirty may, in fact, be safe to drink. You simply can't tell without testing it. When you're in a situation where you can't test it, you can't be sure, so the only safe thing to do is to treat it.

Once you have found a safe place to settle, you'll need a stable supply of water for drinking, cooking, and washing. The source can be a spring, well, stream, or lake. If you have a choice of sources, choose the clearest water, since it will require the least amount of work to purify.

The water from a spring or well is naturally filtered by the earth. It usually requires no further purification, unless it has been polluted by runoff from biological, chemical, or radiological contaminants. Test the water before using it the first time, and cover the spring or well to protect the water from any potential surface contamination.

You can install a pump to draw water from a well or draw it by hand with a bucket and rope. Build a storage tank in case the well runs dry or the pump breaks. If you have a pump, try to keep a spare pump and spare parts on hand. Keep all containers and piping sanitary.

If you are going to use water from another source, you'll need to construct a purification system, running the water through filters that remove progressively smaller particles. As the final step, the water is chemically treated to remove any remaining biological contaminants.

1. Screen the intake pipe at the water source to filter out large debris. Include a reservoir ahead of the filters to allow large particles to settle out of the water before it flows through the system.

2. Allow the water to flow through a filtering system of smaller and smaller stones, using either gravity or a pump.
    a. top layer – coarse rock
    b. next layer – fine rock
    c. next layer – coarse gravel
    d. next layer – fine gravel
    e. bottom layer – sand

The dirtier the water, the more layers you need and the thicker the layers need to be. The layers can be in a single container, or you can have separate containers for each grade of rock. The containers that hold the rocks and sand can be made of any non-toxic non-porous material, such as a 55-gallon drum. You can also use a swimming pool filter as part of your system.

3. Transfer the water to a holding tank. The storage tank should be large enough to hold a week's supply of water. Install the supply outlet several inches above the tank's bottom, and install a drain in the bottom of the tank.

4. Add chlorine to kill bacteria and viruses. Using a do-it-yourself kit, test water from the tap for a concentration of 10 ppm (parts per million) of chlorine. If it tests at a lower concentration, add more chlorine. Test the purity of the water on a regular basis.

The filter will gradually clog, slowing the outflow. You can back-flush with filtered water to clean the layers of rock and sand, but back-flushing mixes the materials together, so you will have to replace the layers of rock and sand periodically.

The delivery system must transport water from the source to the purification system and then to the usage point without picking up dirt or germs.

Camouflage your pipes to prevent an enemy from following them into your compound, and protect your water source and delivery system from poisoning.

Locate livestock, septic systems, solid waste facilities, and chemical storage downhill from your water source to prevent contamination.

Minimize the amount of water you need to purify. Use untreated water for flushing toilets or watering plants.

FOOD

Food: you need to know how to acquire it, how to prepare it, and how to store it.

Food Sources

- Hunt with firearm, bow, spear, or other weapon.
- Trap with a foothold trap, deadfall trap, snare, or other types of traps.
- Fish by hand gathering, hook and line, spear, net, or trap.
- Gather wild edibles, such as berries and mushrooms.
- Cultivate grains, legumes, fruits, and vegetables.
- Raise animals for milk, eggs, honey, and meat.

Food Preparation

If you hunt or trap game, you will have to know how to skin it and butcher it.

If you fish, you will have to know how to scale it, gut it, and fillet it.

Meats and fish are generally safer if thoroughly cooked, since heat destroys bacteria. Fruits and vegetables are generally healthier if eaten raw, but cooking hard foods, such as potatoes or corn, to make them softer can make them easier to eat. If you want to cook food, you will need to have a means to boil it, grill it, bake it, or cook it in some other way.

Food Preservation

If you produce more food than you can consume before it spoils, you will have to preserve it in some way. Many food preservation techniques exist, but it an apocalyptic situation, stick to the simplest ones:

- drying
- salting
- pickling
- canning

Refer to your survival library for a detailed explanation of how to use various food preservation methods.

CLOTHING

Say what you will about Scarlett O'Hara, she was resourceful. When she needed a new dress and no other fabric was available, she yanked down the draperies and fashioned herself a new frock. So it will be with you in an apocalyptic situation, if you are to survive. Besides shelter, you will need clothes to help protect you against cold, heat, rain, snow, hail, windstorms, and sandstorms.

If textile manufacturing breaks down, you will need to not only make your own clothes, but also make your own fabric, using whatever is available, such as:

- animal skins
- fur (from rabbits, squirrels, raccoons, etc.)
- hair (sheep's wool, goat hair, etc.)
- feathers (for garment insulation or bedding)
- tall grass
- broad leaves
- cotton
- flax
- jute
- paper
- rubber

To make cloth from animal or plant fibers, you must first spin the fibers into thread or yarn, and then weave the thread into fabric with a loom or stitch the yarn with knitting needles or a crochet hook to create articles of clothing.

ENERGY

You will need energy in some form to provide:

- power to operate appliances, tools, and equipment
- heat for living space
- heat for water
- heat for cooking
- transportation

Harness the power of the sun, moving water, the wind, plants, fossil fuels, or chemical reactions to serve your needs. Use whatever form of energy is available to produce power:

- photovoltaic panels
- dam
- tide mill
- water wheel
- windmill or wind turbine
- biomass: sugar cane, corn, vegetable oils, animal fats
- wood
- coal
- oil and other petroleum products
- natural gas
- wet-cell or dry-cell batteries

"Baghdad batteries" date from about 200 B. C. If your ancient ancestors were able to figure out how to produce electricity, you can, too.

WASTE TREATMENT

Keep all waste away from your water source.

Sewage

When you're on the move, the proper way to dispose of solid human waste is to bury it.

If you settle in an area without a community sewage treatment facility, you will have to build your own septic system. The simplest form of disposal is to use a pit toilet as a cesspool.

Manure

Keep animal waste away from your living quarters.

Animal dung has several uses:

- ◆ fertilizer
- ◆ fuel (dried like charcoal briquettes, sort of)
- ◆ building material to cement mud bricks together (like mortar)

Compost

In an apocalyptic situation, you will be consuming most of what you find, and you can expect to have very little waste. But if you do have organic matter to dispose of, create a compost pile and use the compost to fertilize a garden. Items suitable for the compost pile:

- ◆ inedible plant fibers, such as stalks, leaves, rinds, peels, corn husks
- ◆ coffee grounds, tea leaves
- ◆ food scraps
- ◆ dead leaves and grass
- ◆ crushed egg shells
- ◆ paper

Do not include animal products, such as meat, eggs, or dairy, since these will attract undesirable wildlife to your compost heap.

SECURITY

If civil law breaks down, you will be on your own to protect yourself and your family.

If the situation warrants it, place sentries at strategic points on your property, and have someone in your group monitor the surveillance cameras. Rotate in shifts to have coverage 24/7.

The point of being a survivalist is to survive. Confrontation should be avoided. To increase your chances of survival, respond to a threat using this sequence:

1. **Retreat.** When threatened by an enemy, retreat if you possibly can.

2. **Negotiate.** If retreating isn't an option, negotiate if you possibly can.

3. **Fight.** If you can't negotiate an agreement, you will have to fight to survive. Engaging an enemy in combat should be a last resort, but if you are forced to fight, fight to win.

WORDS TO LIVE BY

Be as inconspicuous as possible about your emergency preparedness and keep your plans confidential. In the event of widespread shortages, anyone who has stockpiled supplies will become a target of thieves.

Reduce your dependence on the outside world. Move toward the goal of being completely self-sustaining in all areas of survival: water, food, energy, etc. The closer you get to this goal, the more likely you are to survive.

Make safety your top priority. Safety is more important than being on time, avoiding embarrassment, or making money. You can always replace possessions; the only irreplaceable thing is your life.

Anytime you are in doubt about what to do in unfamiliar surroundings, follow the example of the native people or indigenous animals. They have successfully adapted to their environment.

Don't be afraid to fail. If you try something and it doesn't work, try something else!

Cast your net deep, wide, and continuously for resources.

Control the things you can and don't worry about the rest.

And finally, on the last two pages, some ideas to keep you thinking...

Afterword

An emergency is a time for creative thinking. Think about how compound machines use the six simple machines (lever, pulley, wheel and axle, wedge, inclined plane, screw), and how everyday objects can be adapted to meet your needs.

- A playground slide can become a ramp.

- Use dental floss for sewing thread.

- Defrost frozen pipes with a hair dryer.

- Use cat litter to extinguish a small fire.

- Put a piece of chalk in your toolbox to absorb moisture and keep your tools from rusting.

- Use a toothpick to replace a lost screw on your eyeglasses.

- Recycle oil by straining it through a coffee filter.

- Use a wet tea bag as a compress on your gum after a tooth extraction.

- Make a funnel from aluminum foil by rolling it into a cone shape.

- Use brewed tea as a meat tenderizer.

- Tie empty milk jugs together to make a raft.

- Use a straw as an eyedropper.

- Cut holes into a garbage bag to use as a rain slicker.

- Use a clean toilet plunger and bucket as a washtub.

- Cook pasta in a coffee pot and use the spout to drain the water.

- Shave with olive oil in place of shaving cream.

- Make your own saline solution to flush wounds and flush the eyes. Use a heaping teaspoon of table salt per quart of tap water.

Some of the things you can do with a bandana:

- Wear it as a dusk mask.

- Wear it around your neck to protect against sunburn.

- Wear it as a sweatband to keep sweat out of your eyes.

- Wear it wet to cool off in hot weather.

- Wear it around your neck to keep warm in cold weather.

- Wear it as a sling for an injured arm.

- Wear it as an eye patch.

- Use it as a tourniquet.

- Use it as a waist pack.

- Use it to collect berries.

- Use it to filter water.

- Use it as a potholder.

- Use it as a dishcloth or a washcloth.

- Use it as a "help" signal by tying it to the antenna of your car.

- Use it to mark a trail.

- Use it to bind a stone to toss a line over a branch.

- Use it as cordage.

- Use it as a weapon to sling a stone.

- Use it as a wiping cloth to clean and oil firearms.

- Use it as a handkerchief to wipe your runny nose.

Index

Other books in the Survival Series:

Save Your Business!
An Emergency Preparedness and Survival Guide
For Small-Business Owners

Obtain copies of *Survive!* or *Save Your Business!* through:

www.survivalguide.**biz**

or

Blue Peter Enterprises, LLC
P O Box 24755
Dayton, OH 45424

About the Author

I. M. Reddy has 25 years of experience writing for the business market and is a self-taught survivalist.

www.ingramcontent.com/pod-product-compliance
Lightning Source LLC
Chambersburg PA
CBHW050108280326
41933CB00010B/1016